Sheila Cirigiri
Sushil kumar Cirigiri
Venkanna Babu Ghantasala

Understanding Glass Ionomers

Sheila Cirigiri
Sushil kumar Cirigiri
Venkanna Babu Ghantasala

Understanding Glass Ionomers

From Basic Science to Clinical Excellence in Dental Practice

LAP LAMBERT Academic Publishing

Imprint
Any brand names and product names mentioned in this book are subject to trademark, brand or patent protection and are trademarks or registered trademarks of their respective holders. The use of brand names, product names, common names, trade names, product descriptions etc. even without a particular marking in this work is in no way to be construed to mean that such names may be regarded as unrestricted in respect of trademark and brand protection legislation and could thus be used by anyone.

Cover image: www.ingimage.com

Publisher:
LAP LAMBERT Academic Publishing
is a trademark of
Dodo Books Indian Ocean Ltd. and OmniScriptum S.R.L publishing group

120 High Road, East Finchley, London, N2 9ED, United Kingdom
Str. Armeneasca 28/1, office 1, Chisinau MD-2012, Republic of Moldova, Europe
Managing Directors: Ieva Konstantinova, Victoria Ursu
info@omniscriptum.com

Printed at: see last page
ISBN: 978-620-8-43748-0

GLASS IONOMER CEMENTS

CONTENTS

1. INTRODUCTION

Glass ionomer cements (GIC) are one of the most promising restorative materials in dentistry. The unique properties exhibited by GIC attributed for its successful application in dentistry for more than 25years[1].GIC is an unusual material which is neither purely a polymer nor a hydraulic cement but sets by chemical gelation as a reaction between an acid and a base. These unusual properties are probably because they derive their chemistry from silicate cements and zinc polyalkenoic acids from the second.

It is also a kind of composite which can be assumed where its filler particle taking part in setting reaction. It has porcelain like translucency, adheres to tooth substances and have favourable bioactive properties[7]. Translucency is derived from alluminosilicate glass (a base) and adhesive properties are from polyelectorate (an acid).[2]

They bond chemically to dental hard tissues and release fluoride for relatively long period. They exhibit porcelain like translucency with favourable bioactive properties.GIC has very wide range of application in dentistry indeed due to the chemical diversity of two components. Because of which significant advances in technologies and clinical application of GIC can be expected. The GIC has the crucial property of adhering to untreated dentine and enamel which lead to the clinical techniques to minimize the cavity preparation and thus the loss of tooth material. Glass-ionomer is not only bioactive, but has even features of an intelligent material. Glass-ionomer can be called active as it releases fluoride, it can be called intelligent,because it releases fluoride proportionally to the acidity. To some extend it has a pH buffer capacity.[3]

Outside dentistry it has proved useful as a splint/bandage material, a bone cement, a replacement for plaster of paris in slip casting and a model material. Such application have been shown to be very versatile and in recent years they have been subject to the extent that ,at this time, they are really very different from the original ASPA that was first marketed in 1976. [5,6.]

The GIC has come a long way since it was first introduced. It has many versions &various applications too. Can it be developed still further is in question. Though stronger and more aesthetic versions (materials) with improved handling characteristics are now available, lack of toughness remains a problem. Finishing and carvability like amalgam is still a problem with current material. Early moisture contamination and desiccation problems have not been entirely solved. Varnishing of the restoration is still required. The most intractable problems will be overcome is likely to be lack of strength and toughness. Most of these problems will be overcome as development proceeds.[2]

2. SCIENTIFIC AND CLINICAL DEVELOPMENT OF GIC

During early and mid 1960's the science and technology of clinical dental materials remained where they had been almost 60years before. The period of the late 1960's and early 1970's was a most creative one in the development of new materials. The invention of GIC in 1969(first reported by Wilson and Kent in 1971) resulted directly from basic studies on dental silicate cements was replaced by organic chelating acid (Wilson 1968).The silicates were useful because they were never really properly understood; they were badly abused by the profession and never reached their full potential.

It was hoped that following the development of polycarboxylate cements it would be possible to develop another stronger material that would adhere long term to dental structures. The aqueous solution of phosphoric acid was replaced with aqueous solution of polycarboxylic acid and, based on knowledge in glass chemistry, a more reactive glass powder with the biocompatibility and adhesive qualities of a polyacrylic liquid (Wilson &Mclean 1988; Atkinson &Pearson 1985)

Development of GIC is a combination of both scientific and clinical effort . Though its original invention happened in laboratory, but its later development was based on its clinical applicability.

SCIENTIFIC DEVELOPMENT

Scientific development of GIC can be divided into two phases

1. Improving properties to make it practical for anterior restorations.

2. Modifying properties in order to extend its range of applications.

Wilson in 1965 &1966 worked on cements by mixing silicate glass powder with aqueous solutions of various organic acids including polyacrylic acid. Later Wilson along with Kent and Lewis in 1968&69 employed novel glass formulations for producing hydrolytically stable cements. They observed that setting of these cements was controlled by alumina /silica ratio in the glass. The first GIC lacked workability and hardened slowly. In (1973, 1979) Kent et al substituted a glass called (G.200) which was rich in fluoride which gave a usable cement called alumino silicate polyacrylate-I(ASPA-1)

Scientific	Clinical
Original invention, ASPA I: 1969 (Wilson & Kent, 1971, 1972, 1973)	First clinical trials: 1970 (McLean)
First practical material: ASPA II: 1972 (Wilson & Crisp, 1976)	
First marketable material, ASPA IV: 1973 (Crisp & Wilson, 1977) (Europe 1975, Australia 1976, USA 1977)	Class I restorations, fissure sealing, preventive dentistry (McLean & Wilson, 1974)
Luting agent, ASPA IVa: 1975 (Wilson et al., 1977)	Erosion lesions, deciduous teeth, lining, luting, composite/ionomer laminates (McLean & Wilson, 1977a, 1977b, 1977c)
Improved translucency, ASPA X: 1977 (Crisp, Abel, & Wilson, 1979)	Improved clinical techniques: 1976-1977 (Mount & Makinson, 1978)
	Approximal lesions, minimal cavity preparation (buccal approach) (McLean 1980)
Silver-tin alloy, metal oxide and carbon-reinforced cements: 1977 (Sced & Wilson, 1980; Simmons, 1983)	
Cermet ionomer cements: 1978 (McLean & Glasser, 1985)	
Water-activated cements, ASPA V: 1982 (Prosser et al., 1984)	Water-activated luting agent (McLean et al., 1984; Prosser et al., 1984)
	Tunnel Class I and II pr-eparations (Hunt, 1984; Knight, 1984; McLean, 1986)
	Double-etch ionomer/composite-rein laminates (McLean et al., 1985)

These cements had sluggish set, less working time and due to high fluoride opaque G-200 glass gave cement with translucency below that required for general clinical use. The key discovery was by Wilson & crisp in 1972 (reported in 1976) who found that tartaric acid modified the cement forming reaction which improved manipulation, extended working time and sharpening the setting rate. This development of ASPA I was termed as ASPA II and constituted the first practical GIC. After the advent of ASPA II though the hardening and vulnerability to water was comparatively less than ASPA I, its set was still sluggish and aesthetics were not good as compared to present standards. later physical properties were recently improved. Initially another disadvantage was the tendency of the liquid to gel. Crisp et.al (1975) solved this problem by developing and copolymer of acrylic and itaconic acid that did not gel at high concentrations in aqueous solution. this was called as ASPA IV. However ASPA-IV was found to be inferior to ASPA II in other properties. Many studies were going on during that period for exploring the adhesive properties of GIC. Later McLean and Wilson (1977) stated that this material was ideal for Class V erosion lesion. its development helped in accomplishing the prevention of doubtful technique of extending cavities by mechanical preparation.

By 1979 Crisp et.al developed ASPA X which had good clinical results and excellent transluscency. The luting version of GIC which had fine grain version was developed by Wilson et.al for the first time in 1977 as was called ASPA IVa . McLean and Wilson in a review of the state of the art and forecast of the future clinical developments of GIC stated a variety of clinical applications, suggested the use in pediatric dentistry and as a liner in composite resin/ionomer laminates which is only recently adopted . Minimal cavity preparation was clearly enunciated .

Though the findings of these papers which are valid today were discovered very early unfortunately they were ignored for many years. The further development was emphasized in improvement of the instability of polyacrylic solutions. It was described much before by Wilson and Kent (1973) that developing special copolymers which although stable in water but cant yield best cements will not solve the problem . Instead these authors reported the use of polyacrylic acid in dry powder form blended with glass powder. This cement was formed by mixing with water or tartaric acid solutions. This resulted in the development of ASPA V(Posser et.al1984)

After discovery of ASPA V many problems were solved, for example ASPA IV a. a luting cements with a low viscosity polyacid liquid which lacked the mobility of traditional Zn phosphate cement. But ASPA Va had another advantage was that higher concentrations higher molecular weight can be used which results in cements of higher strength.

The concept of minimal cavity preparations has undergone steady development over the years. The first application of this concept was the simple opening of class I carious lesions or early approximal lesions involving a buccal or lateral marginal ridge approach (McLean,1980). The idea has been extended using tunnel preparation for class II carious lesions.(Hunt 1984,Knight,McLean 1986).Later in 1980-1983 Sced, Wilson and Simmons attempted to improve the strength of GIC by incorporating metallic oxide and metal alloy fillers Mclean and Gasser (1985) made a major advancement in improving wear resistance by fusing silver particles onto the ionomer glass giving the cement radioopacity , burnishability and smoother surfaced material with concomitant advantages.[2]

Moore et.al(1985) have reported that resistance to abrasion is improved considerably. These new cermets have been subsequently developed for clinical use.(Mclean 1986). GIC'S are not however recommended for restorations where toughness and resistance to occlusal contact is adequate.(Mclean 1980).it has generally been recognized that GIC wear resistance to occlusal contact is inadequate. Clinical studies have shown that gradual loss of contour can be expected because of surface wear and chemical degradation (Smales and Joyce1978) . one study of commercial GIC, with a commercial resin composite as a control found that the GIC,with a commercial resin composite as a control found that the GIC abraded about 3 times more by volume than did the composite (Mclean1984).the addition of silver alloy powder to GIC in particular results in a number of physical property improvements (CROLL-1990).the silver cermet material has a light grey color has a major disadvantage in that it has a low fracture toughness making it of limited value in regions subjected to occlusal stresss (McLean and Gasser1985).silver released from cermet can diffuse into surrounding structures and cause discoloration (sarkar et.al:1988and Philips 1986) GIC'S, including cermets ,are technique sensitive (Knibbs and Plant 1986;Smales and gerke; Watson 1990). Poor quality GIC restorations are not uncommon , although technique sensitivity is not a problem that often finds it way into the dental literature . although GICs exhibit significantly less polymerization shrinkage than do composites,some curing contraction does generally occur,leading to marginal gap formation(Feltzier etal 1988;saunders etal 1990).

3. COMPOSITION

Definition:

A. GIC is an acid-base reaction cement as defined by Wilson (1978) and Wygant (1958), the product of reaction being a hydrogel salt which acts as a binding matrix (Alan D. Wilson, GIC).

B. According to Skinners – Glass ionomer is the generic name of a group of materials that use silicate glass powder and an aqueous solution of polyacrylic acid. Also known as "Polyalkenoate cement".

C. A cement that consists of a basic glass and an acidic polymer which sets by an acid base reaction between these components as described by Wilson and Nicholson (QI vol. 25 No. 9, 1994).

The GICs are probably more accurately and scientifically known as glass alkeonate cements. The composition of GIC are complex and varied . no two commercial examples are chemically identical and they may even differ qualitatively.

As defined by Wilson and Wygnat (1958) the GIC is an acid base reaction cement i.e it can be called as true acid base materials where the base is a flouro alumino silicate glass with a high fluoride cement and this interacts polyalkenoic acid. The product of this reaction is a hydrogel salt which acts as a binding matrix. The complex and varied nature of GIC is because of its composition which has the basic component, which is a glass (calcium alumino silicate glass) containing fluoride and acid is a polyelectrolyte, which is a homopolymer or copolymer of unsaturated carboxylic acids which are alkeonic in nature.

Many hundreds of glasses have been prepared in the U.K's laboratory of the Government chemist by A.D Wilson and his coworkers and many alkeonic acids are known but polyacrylic acid being the most commonly used .Chemical diversity of the two materials being immune provide much scope for new formulations which can be used for specific applications.[5,6]

GLASSES:

The composition of the glass has a large variations of which the ion leachable calcium alumino silicates are the only ones which have practical applications. The chemical composition of the original ionomer glass ,G-200 is as follows: as given by Barry et.al 1978.

Chemical composition of the original ionomer glass, G-200 :

Species	Composition (%)
SiO_2	30.1
Al_2O_3	19.9
AlF_3	2.6
CaF_2	34.5
NaF	3.7
$AlPO_4$	10.0

The three essential constituents of dental ionomer glasses are silica, calcium fluoride and alumina. Glasses are prepared by fusing the components between 1100*C and 1500*c i.e the exact temperature of fusion depends on the chemical makeup of the fusion mixture. Later the melted components are poured onto metal plate or into water.

Then the glass is ground to fine powder where maximum particle size for restorative cements being 50 micrometers and 20 micrometers for luting cements. The finer the particle size the stronger the cemet and rapid the setting reaction.

The visual appearance of the glass whether it is clear ,opal or opaque depends on the composition. Glasses high in silica (i.e greater than 40% are transparent, whereas glasses high in calcium fluoride or alumina are opaque. The opaqueness is due to presence of dispersed crystalline phases of fluorite or corundum such a composition might better be described as glass ceramic rather than a glass.

The formation of cement is also related to glass composition. The alumina:silica ratio of the glass is crucial and required to be 1:2 or more by mass for cement formation [Wilson et.al,Kent et.al(1980)]. This ratio will allows replacement of silicon by aluminium which render network susceptible to acid attack. Thus with increase in the ratio of alumina/silica gives rise to glasses even more basic and reactive which will have lower setting times of the cements. However limit is reached when alumina/silica ratio will not effect the setting time;or it may be slightly prolonged. But the nature of the glass changes from being clear to opaque as corundum separates out from the glass.

Apart from the setting time and opacity the other properties affected are;compressive strengths increases with increase alumina content but the transluscency of the glass decreases. The ionomer glasses are different from most of the silicate glasses as they are decomposed for the cement formation . But why does the cement forming propensity of dental ionomer glasses derive from their decomposition in the presence of acids?

The reason lies in the structure of the glass. A silica glass is a highly crosslinked network of connected silicon and oxygen atoms. It does not carry an electric charge, and is impervious to acid attack. By contrast, the ionomer glass is an ionic polymer–the network is similar to that of silica, but it contains negative sites because aluminium has partly replaced silicon in the glass network. Aluminium can enter the silica network, replacing silicon, thus conferring a negative charge on the network, which becomes basic and susceptible to attack by hydrogen ions from the acid.

If there are enough aluminium atoms in the network, all of the connecting links in the network will be broken down and the glass will be completely decomposed. Such a glass has cement-forming potential. Thus Al_2O_3/SiO_2 ratio of the glass is crucial as it determines whether the glass network will break down at all when exposed to acids, and the rate at which the breakdown occurs. Glasses used in practice are generally more complex than the simple three-component systems. And the fluxing action of calcium fluoride is generally supplemented by the addition of cryolite (Na_3AlF_6). This flux reduces the temperature at which the glass will fuse and increases the translucency of the set cement. Aluminium phosphate is also often included in the glass fusion mixtures; it too improves translucency and apparently adds body to the cement paste.

Barry and coworkers (1979)were probably the one who did research on glass structure.The glass studied by Barry et al., was G-200, the basis of the first practical glass-ionomer cement, but not typical of present-day ionomer glasses. The G-200 contains phase-separated glass droplets of complex structure, as well as massive inclusions of fluorite.

More recently, studies (Hill and Wilson, 1986) indicate that other opal glasses, while not containing inclusions of fluorite, do contain droplets similar to those in G-200. These phase-separated droplets are calcium-rich (compared with the continuous-phase) and contain a crystalline core of calcium and fluoride surrounded by an amorphous phase rich in calcium but containing some aluminium and silicon. This amorphous phase is selectively leached by acids. Thus calcium is preferentially leached by acids from the glass.

Treatment of glasses :

Washing glasses with mineral or organic acids has been advocated in order to reduce the concentration of calcium at the surface of phase-separated droplets in the glass. This process reduces the amount of calcium extracted during the early stages of the reaction, and so prolongs working time (Schmitt et al., 1981a).

Effect of particle size on cement properties :

Glass composition has a considerable effect on cement properties. Indeed, for a glass to have cement-forming properties at all, it must fulfill certain basic requirements. Glass composition affects working characteristics, setting time, and resistance to erosion, aesthetics, and cement strength. In addition, the presence of phase-separated droplets will affect both cement translucency and strength.

Another important factor is the particle size of the glass powder. It is obvious that, other things being equal, the finer the particle size (i.e., the greater the specific surface of the powder), the faster the setting reaction will be. Data are not available for the glass-ionomer cements, but the research of Kent and Wilson (1971), who studied the effect of particle size on dental silicate cement properties, confirms this observation. These researchers also found that, other things being equal, fine-grained glasses produced the strongest cements. To achieve the film thickness of 20 μm demanded of a luting agent, a fine-grained glass has to be used (Wilson et al., 1977b). The tendency over the years has been for finer-grained powders to be used in restorative materials.

Disperse-phase glasses :

Glasses may be modified by phase separation. Wilson and coworkers (1980) observed that clear glasses yielded weaker cements than glasses containing droplets of a disperse phase. The observation led Prosser and coworkers (1986) to increase deliberately the amount of the disperse phase in a glass: they found that when this was done the flexural strength of the cements was increased. Suitable disperse phases were found to be corundum, rutile (TiO_2), baddeleyite (ZrO_2), and tieilite (Al_2TiO_5). Baddeleyite has been found in one commercial core material. [4,10]

Fibre reinforcement :

The incorporation of alumina fibres and other fibres (Sced and Wilson, 1980) has been used to improve flexural strength of glass-ionomer cements-50 MPa can be obtained but apparently abrasion resistance is poor.

Effect of phase-separated crystallites on cement strength :

Glass	Phase-separated crystallites	Flexural strength (MPa)
G.228	None	21
G-309	Fluorite (GaF_2) Corundum (Al_2O_3)	33
G-385	Rutile (TiO_2) Tieilite (Al_2TiO_5)	30
G-318	Baddeleyite (ZrO_2)	28

Effect of reinforcing filers on flexural strength of glass-ionomer cements :

Filler	Filler/glass ratio (by mass)	Flexural strength (MPa)
None	-	10
Silica fibre	1:2	26
Glass fibre	1:2	21
G-200 Glass fibre	1.4:1	30
Carbon fibre	1:4	53
Alumina fibre	1:3	44
Ag_3Sn	4.5:1	40
Ag_3Sn_5	4.5:1	13

Metallic inclusions:

Sced and Wilson (1980) found that the amalgam alloys could be incorporated into glass-ionomer cements and that these served to increase the flexural strength. These systems have been used clinically by Simmons (1983) and are available commercially. However, their aesthetics are poor and they do not take burnish. Their resistance to abrasion is also less than that of regular glass-ionomer cements (Moore et al., 1985).[11]

Cermet-ionomer cements :

In an attempt to improve the abrasion resistance and strength of glass-ionomer cements. McLean and Gasser (1985) developed the cermet-ionomer cements. These cements, unlike simple mixtures of alloy particles or metal fibres, contain glass-metal powders sintered to high density that can be made to reach with poly-acids to form a cement. Ion-leachable calcium fluoroaluminosilicate glasses are used in the preparation of the glass powder. The set cement can be burnished or polished to produce a metal finish but the surface will not be comparable to the typical Beilby veneer of metals.

Any of the precious metals well known in dentistry may be used in the preparation of these cements, but gold and silver are the most suitable. The glass-metal powder is compressed in a pelletizer; palletizing is preferably carried out at high pressures in a hydraulic press (usually at pressures above 300 MPa). It is favourable to evacuate the pelleting chamber during palletizing at pressures around 100 MPa. The compressed pellets are then fused at around 800^0C. The sintered metal-glass composite, when ground to a fine powder, retains its characteristics because the metal powder remains firmly bonded in the glass. It is interesting to note that the ground powder is more rounded than a conventionally ground glass powder, which imparts to the cement the excellent handling properties of high packing density and low porosity.

At present a commercial cermet-ionomer cement is available that contains fine silver powder particles of less than 3.5 µm in size. Colour has also been improved by the addition of up to 5% titanium dioxide.

Physical properties:

By fusing silver powder into the glass, very strong bonding of the metal has been achieved allowing the surface to be burnished which in turn has dramatically improved abrasion resistance. McKinney and coworkers (1986) considered that the silver has a lubricating effect on the surface, and McLean and Gasser (1985) suggested that the sintered metal powder was lowering the coefficient of friction. This would appear to be borne out by clinical trails.The flexural strength of the cermet-cements is marginally better than the best glass-ionomer cements but as yet cannot be compared in strength to composite resins and amalgam alloys. They are therefore unsuitable for use in a high-stress-bearing cavity such as a large Class II lesion.

Polyelectrolytes :

Polyelectrolytes are interesting substances, which, as their name implies, are both electrolytes and polymers. The notion that polymers are soluble in water is an unusual one, but such substances are of considerable biological importance.

The polyelectrolytes used in glass-ionomer cements can be described as poly(alkenoic acids); indeed, the international organization for standardization name for glass-ionomer cement that contains polyelectrolytes is glass polyalkenoate cement. These polyacids include the homopolymers or copolymers of unsalurated mono-, di-, and tri-carboxylic acids, particularly those of acrylic acid (Crisp et al., 1980b). The more important carboxylic acids in the ionomer system include acrylic acid, maleic acid, and itaconic acid. The numbers of homopolymers and copolymers that can be built from these three structural units of different configurations and molecular weights is considerable.

The polyacid may be either in the form of a concentrated aqueous solution (40% to 50% by mass) or blended dry with the glass powder, when the system is activated by mixing with either water or an aqueous solution of tartaric acid (McLean et al., 1984).

The most important of the polyacids used to date have been the poly(acrylic acids) themselves, copolymers of acrylic and itaconic acids (Crisp et al., 1980b), and copolymers or acrylic and maleic acids (Schmitt et al., 1981b). There are differences in functionality and acid strength between these polyacids. Poly(maleic acid) contains twice as many carboxyl groups as poly(acrylic acid) and is a stronger acid. It would be expected to be more reactive and required less reactive glasses than those used in combination with poly(acrylic acid).

Composition of experimental ASPA cements:

Cement	**Class**	**Type**	**Powder**	**Liquid**
ASPA I	Conventional	Filling	G-200	50% PA-1
ASPA II	Conventional	Filling	G-200	47.5% PA-1, 5% TTA
ASPA III	Conventional	Filling	G-200	45.0% PA-1, 5% TTA, 5% CH_3OH
ASPA IV	Conventional	Filling	G-200	47.5% PA-48, 5% TTA
ASPA IVa	Conventional	Luting	G-200a	47.5% PA-48, 5% TTA
ASPA V	Water-hardening	Filing	G-200: G-200a:	10% TTA
ASPA Va	Water-hardening	Luting	G-200a: PA-2 (2.5:1)	10% TTA
ASPA X	Conventional	Filling	G-338	47.5% PA-48, 5% TTA

Key	
G-200	Glass powder: maximum grain size 50 μm, composition: 29.0% SiO_2, 16.5% Al_2O_3, 7.3% AlF_3, 34.3% CaF_2, 3.0% NaF, 9,9% $AlPO_4$ (Kent et al., 1979).
G-200a	Glass powder: maximum grain size 15 μm, composition: G-200 (Wilson et al., 1977b).
TTA	(+)-tartaric acid.
PA-1	Poly(acrylic acid) NW(wt. avg.) = 23,000 (Crisp et al., 1980b)
PA-2	Poly(acrylic acid) MW(wt. avg.) = 50,000 (Crisp et al., 1980b)
PA-48	Acrylic acid/itaconic acid 2:1 copolymer MW(wt. avg.) = 10,400 (Crisp et al., 1980b)

The first practical glass-ionomer cement. ASPA II, used poly(acrylic acid) as the cement-forming acid. However, this system was not suitable for marketing because a 50% solution of poly(acrylic acid) will gel after a period of time as the result of a slow increase in hydrogen bonding (Crisp et al., 1975). Poly(acrylic acid) chains are flexible and are constantly changing their configurations; when segments of a pair of chains approach each other, an intermolecular hydrogen bond can be formed. This is a slow but continuing process, which is, in effect, slowly cross-linking poly(acrylic acid). It ultimately reduces solubility, causing gelation[4,5,6].

One approach adopted by Wilson and Crisp (1974) was to add methyl alcohol to poly(acrylic acid) solutions as an agent that inhibits the ordering of structures in solution. This glass ionomer cement was known as ASPA III. Although the gelation of poly(acrylic acid) was prevented, McLean found that the cement stained in the mouth. Another approach had to be adopted.[4,5,6]

Crisp and Wilson (1977) reasoned that copolymers of acrylic acid with other unsaturated carboxylic acids would be less regular than simple poly(acrylic acid) and so less liable to form intermolecular hydrogen bonds. They synthesized a copolymer of acrylic and itaconic acid which proved indefinitely stable in a 50% aqueous solution. This copolymer was used in ASPA IV, which was otherwise identical to ASPA II. A commercial glass-ionomer cement was based on the ASPA IV formula[4,5,6].

It would be expected that different molecular configurations would affect adhesion; recent evidence supports this hypothesis. Aboush and Jenkins (1986) have shown that cements based on poly(acrylic acid) bond more strongly to enamel and dentine than to cements based on copolymers of acrylic acid with itaconic or maleic acid. Another difference, noted by Setchell and coworkers (1985), is that cements based on copolymers of acrylic and maleic acids are apparently less resistant to acid attack than those based on poly(acrylic acid), a result confirmed by Wilson and coworkers (1986). But these cements are harder than those of poly(acrylic acid), which aids early finishing (Mount and Makinson, 1982; Matis and Philips, 1986). This can be attributed to a more highly cross-linked matrix arising from the greater number of carboxyl groups. [4,5,6]

The molecular weight (relative molar mass) and the concentration of the polyacid affects cement strength. increases in either will shorten set time and increase the strength of the set time and increase the strength of the set cement (Wilson et al., 1977a; Prosser et al., 1986; Crisp et al., 1977).

Since strength is a welcome attribute, such modifications would appear desirable. when the polyacid is present in solution, an increase in either molecular weight or concentration will increase the viscosity of the liquid, making the cement pastes progressively more difficult to manipulate. Hence, there is a trend away from using polyacid in solution and toward using it in dry solid form for blending with the glass powder. The liquid for cement formation is then either plain water or an aqueous solution of tartaric acid, both of low viscosity. In this system the molecular weight and effective polyacid concentration can be increased, to some extent, without rendering the pasts unworkable. Thus, this type of glass-ionomer cement tends to be stronger than the other.

Effect of the nature of the poly(alkenoic acid) on cement properties[4,12] :

From the previous discussion it is apparent that the nature of the polyacid does have some effect on cement properties, although this is less marked than in the case with glass composition. The type of polyacid used is though to affect setting time, and its molecular weight affects strength. The higher the molecular weight of the polyacid, the higher will be the strength of the cement. However, against this is the increasing viscosity of the mix, which limits the molecular weight of the polyacid employed.

Water

Water is often not considered a constituent of glass-ionomer cement, but it is, in fact, a very important one. It is the reaction medium and also plays a role in hydrating reaction products, that is, metal poly(alkenoate) salts and silica gel. Attempts to replace it even partially with another solvent, such as alcohol gives rise to very weak cement (Hornsby, 1977).

Too much water in the system results in weak, slow-setting cements. Some reduction in the amount of water is beneficial: cements set faster and are stronger and more durable. However, once this optimum limit is reached, there is insufficient water for the reaction and for hydration-the result is a weakening of the cement (Prosser et al., 1986).

Tartaric acid [14]:

In their early studies, Wilson and Kent (1973) found that the principal obstacle to developing a practical glass-ionomer cement was the sluggish nature of the set. Working time was minimal and hardening was slow. The future of the system appeared doubtful. However, they found that one or two glasses exceptionally high in fluoride were capable of reaching the minimal acceptable setting characteristic. Even so, these cements set sluggishly and had low translucency because of the large amounts of fluorite crystallites in the glasses. The simple two component glass plus polyacid does not constitute an adequate system.

For this reason, a search was made for additives to control the setting reaction, and in 1976 Wilson and coworkers reported that tartaric acid was extremely effective. Depending on the nature of the glass, the working time is unaffected or even prolonged, and the setting rate is markedly increased (Wilson and Crisp, 1976; Wilson et al., 1976; [Cook], 1983; Crisp and Wilson, 1976; Prosser et al., 1982). The addition of tartaric acid made the glass-ionomer cement system a practical one. It enabled the fluoride content of the glasses to be reduced, an important step in the production of clear or slightly opal glasses, which form the basis of glass-ionomer cements with enhanced translucency. In addition, the number of glasses that could be used for cement formation was increased dramatically.

Rheological studies show that tartaric acid delays the onset of viscosity, and that the greater the concentration of tartaric acid, the longer the delay (Cook, 1983; Hill and Wilson, 1986).

The action of tartaric acid is apparently unique. Other-rate-controlling additives are known, but even other hydroxycarboxylic acids do not have the unique delaying effect of tartaric acid-even mesotartaric acid is ineffective (Crisp et al., 1979). Only the positive enantiomorph of tartaric acid produces the desired effect[13].

Other additives :

Other additives are used to control the setting reaction of glass-ionomer cements but they either accelerate the set at the expense of working time or vice versa (Wilson et al., 1976; Tomioka et al., 1983; Crisp et al., 1980a). Polyphosphates can be used to extend working time but the set is prolonged. Certain metal salts, such as stannous fluoride, accelerate setting but reduce working time. All are useful only if used in conjunction with (+)-tartaric acid.

Packaging and dispensing :

As we have seen, the modern glassionomer cement has four constituents: glass, polyacid, tartaric acid, and water. The material is presented to the clinician as a two-component powder/liquid pack.

In the older, conventional form, the powder was simply ground glass, and the liquid contained the polyacid and tartaric acid in solution. More recently a new presentation has appeared-the so-called water-hardening cements-where the polyacid is dried and mixed with the glass to form a powder blend (Prosser et al., 1984; McLean et al., 1984). The liquid is then either water (in which case dried tartaric acid is incorporated into the powder blend) or a solution of tartaric acid.

The term "anhydrous cement" has been inappropriately applied to these materials. They are water-based cements, with water playing an essential role in both the reaction and the cement structure. Zinc oxide-eugenol cements, where eugenol is the reaction medium, are the true anhydrous cements[4]

Types :

Apart from the different packaging just described, glass-ionomer cements come in many forms. They are best distinguished by usage.

Type 1: luting agents

Flow properties and minimal film thickness are essential in cements used as luting agents. Fine-grained glass powders with maximum grain sizes of 15 µm or less are employed. Some clinicians require radio-opacity, which can be obtained by replacing calcium in the glass with strontium or lanthanum. When translucency is not required, phase-separated glass, a cermet ionomer, or a glass combined with zinc oxide can be used.

Type II: aesthetic filling materials

In anterior restorations, where aesthetics is important, adequate translucency is required of a glass ionomer cement. Phase-separated glass or cermet ionomers cannot be used. Clear glasses tend to have high silica/alumina ratios, and cements formed from them tend to harden slowly.

Type II: bis-reinforced filling materials

This category covers the cermet (glass-metal) derivatives of type II materials. These are not aesthetic but are more resistant to abrasion.

Type III: lining, base, and fissure-sealing materials

Strength and radiopacity are important when a glass-ionomer cement is to be used as a lining, base, or fissure sealant. Fine-grained glasses are often employed when translucency is not important. Some lining materials contain zinc oxide, which tends to buffer the system and render the cement radio-opaque. These are useful properties, but are obtained at the price of some loss of strength. Cermet-ionomer cements can also be used. The Type III classification could well be extended to include nonaesthetic glassionomer materials. Some of these materials set very quickly because they are used in the "double laminate" or "sandwich" technique.

Pit and fissure sealants :

One manufacturer makes a special high fluoride cement for use as a pit and fissure sealant. The original G-200 was, of course, a high-fluoride glass.

Type I and Type II materials have national and international specifications under the Bristish Standards Institution (BS) and the International Standards Organization (ISO):

BS 6039:1981/Glass-Ionomer Cements

ISO 7489:1986/Glass-Polyalkenoate Cements

Type III is included in the ISO Draft Proposal for Dental Cements.

Although versions of the glass-ionomer cement are marketed specifically for pit and fissure sealing, such materials could well be included in the Type I classification

Commercial materials :

Leading commercial materials that are, or have been, on the market are listed in Table. All materials are based on fluoroaluminosilicate glasses; many of them are qualitatively similar to G-200. More recent glasses, however, tend to contain more sodium and less fluoride.

Unlike G-200, some glasses used in Type II formulations are clear, which is one of the reasons why many modern glass-ionomer cements have improved translucency.

However, glasses used in Type I cements frequently contain fluorite crystallites (CaF_2) and are thus opal. Although this adversely affects the translucency of the cements these glasses impart favourable setting and strength qualities to the cement.

Radiopacity is found in some materials. This is attained by incorporating strontium, barium or lanthanum into the glass composition, fusing silver to the glass, or mixing in zinc oxide. Current glass-ionomer cements use a variety of polyacids-poly (acrylic acid), copolymers of acrylic acid with maleic acid-to increase reactivity, with itaconic acids for greater stability in aqueous solutions, and with tricarballylic acid. Tannic acid is found in some compositions in order to enhance bonding to dentine because tannic acid adheres to collagen. The polyacid can be present as a solution or added to the glass powder as a dry solid.

All varieties of cement contain (+)-tartaric acid to modify the setting reaction. Sometimes other additives are employed as well, for example, the polyphosphates or tetrahydrofuranetetracarboxylic acid. [4]

Major brands of glass-ionomer cement :

Name	Type	Manufacturer
De Trey Aspa	II	Amalgamated dental Co., Weybridge, England
Chembond	I	
Chem-Fil	II	Dentsply international Inc.,
Aqua-Cem	I	Weybridge, England, and York, Pa.
Chem-Fil II	II	
Chem-Fil II	II	
Chem-Fil Express	II	
Chem-Fil Junior	II	
Ketac-Fil	II	
Chelon	II	
Ketac-Cem	I	
Ketac-Cem Radio-opaque	I, Radio-opaque	ESPE GmbH, Seefeld/Oberbay, west Germany, and Valley Stream, N.Y.
Ketac-Bond	III	
Ketac-Silver	II cermet	
Chelon-Silver	II Cermet	
Fuji lonomer I	I	
Fuji lonomer II	II	
Fuji Lining	III lining	G-C International Corp., Tokyo,
Fuji lonomer III	Pit and fissure	And Scottsdale, Ariz.
Fuji Miracle Mix	Amalgam filled	
Glas-lonomer Type I	I	
Glas-lonomer Type II	II	Shofu Dental corp., Kyoto, Japan, and Menlo Park, Calif.
Glas-lonomer Base	III	
Shofu Lining	III	

4. CLASSIFICATION

A. According to Wilson and Mclean (1988)

Type I : Luting cements

Type II : Restorative cements

- Aesthetic Restorative
- Reinforced Restorative

Type III: Fast setting lining materials and fissure sealants

B. According to application

Type I : Luting cements

Type II : Restorative cements

Type III : Liner and Bases

Type IV : Core build up

Type V : Orthodontic cement

Type VI : Fissure sealant

Newer Classification

1. Traditional GIC

a. Type I : Luting

b. Type II : Restorative

c. Type III : Liners and Bases

2. Metal modified Glass Ionomer

a. Miracle mix
b. Cermet

3. Light cure GIC

4. Hybrid Glass Ionomer (RMGIC)

a. Composite resin in which fillers substituted with glass particles
b. Pre cured glasses blended into composites

1. **According to manufacturers GC Fuji**

Fuji I	: Luting
Fuji II	: Restorative
Fuji III	: Fissure protection
Fuji lining	: Liner
Fuji Ortho	: Ortho bonding
Fuji VII	: Pit & fissure sealant
Fuji VIII	: Anterior Esthetic (ART)
Fuji IX	: ART High strength
Fuji IX GP	: Condensable

By Skinners

A. Type I – Luting cements.

Type II – Restorative materials.

Type III – Liners and base.

Type IV – Metal reinforced - Miracle mix

- Cermet

Type IX – For geriatric and pediatric patients.

B. By Wilson and Mclean 1988a; Mount 1989a (Based on application) (Opt. Dents, 1994).

Type I – Luting crowns, bridges and orthodontic brackets.

Type II – Restorative cements.

Type II 1 – Esthetic restoration cements.

Type II 2 – Reinforced restoration cements.

Type III - Lining cements with powder / liquid ratio 1.5: 1.

- Dentine substitute or base with powder / liquid ratio 3:1.

According Mclean etal 1994

Type I – Luting:

Use: Cementation of crowns, bridges, inlays, orthodontic appliances
Setting rate: Fast set
Powder: liquid ratio: 1.5:1
Radiopaque: Generally
Film thickness: $< 20\ \mu m$

Type II: Restorative
Type II.1: Restorative Aesthetic

Use: Aesthetic restorations
Setting rate: Auto cure - slow resistance to water uptake
Resin modified: Fast set, immediate resistane to water uptake
P : L : 3:1 or greater
Radiopaque: Most materials

Type II.2: Restorative Reinforced
Use: Where increased physicalproperties are required but aesthics is not important
Setting rate: Fast set
P : L : 3:1 or greater
Radiopaque: Always

Type III: Lining or Bases

Lining:
Use: in thin section as thermal barrier under metal restorations
Setting rate: Fast set
P : L : 1.5:1
Base
Use: in combination with composite resin in laminate technique
Setting rate:Fast set
P : L ; 3:1 or greater
Radiopaque: Always

Hickel's Classification:

To create a clearly structured classification for tooth colored plastic restorative materials Hickel suggested assigning the materials to classes corresponding to their water content as possible acid-base reaction during setting

Glass Ionomer cements	**Resin composites**
(Water based)	(No water added)
Conventional	Hybrid composites
Metal-reinforced (Cermet)	Microfilled
Highly viscous	Ormocers
Resin modified (Hybrid ionomers)	Compomer

Traditional Classification: Application oriented:

Type I: For luting inlays, onlays, crowns and bridges, has a film thickness upto 20 μm or less

Type II: For restorations in low stress bearing areas. Film thickness upto 45 μm

Type III: For sealing pits and fissures,film thickness 25-35 μm

Type IV: includes metal-reinforced ionomers, used for high stress bearing areas. Film thickness 45 μm & over

Type V: Light cured glass ionomers.

Classification by use:

Eight classes are formed

1. Glass ionomer luting cements are used as luting agents, auto cure
2. Glass Ionomer Restoratives: used as restorative materials, available in more shades, high filler load, much higher film thickness, auto cured
3. Glass-metal Ionomer mixtures: are intended for bases and build ups (Admixtures)
4. Cermet-Ionomers: Ionomers containing metal-fused to glass particles. Neither the glass metal nor the Cermet ionomers are tooth colored, Auto cre.
5. Glass Ionomer Liners: Rapid setting radiopaue materials for dentin liners under composites and amalgam, Light Cured
6. Glass Ionomer Bases: Bases under other restoratives. These materials are generally stringer but sometimes pulpally compatible than lining cements. Stress bearing situations, Auto cured
7. Glass Ionomer Sealants: for sealing pits and fissures. Auto Cured
   Resin modified Glass Ionomer: Light and Dual cured Glass Ionomers

Types of conventional glass-ionomer cements

Glass-ionomers are currently used for various clinical applications. A large number of products are available, each with a more or less different formulation to fulfill the required characteristics for a specific field of application.

Glass-ionomers for direct restoration

The first glass-ionomer cement developed for filling was called Alumino Silicate Poly-Acrylate (ASPA; Dentsply). Currently, many glass-ionomer products are available for restorative purposes. Although resin based composites possess superior mechanical properties and better esthetics than glass-ionomer cements, composite resins require bonding agents because they are usually hydrophobic and thus do not adhere well to teeth. Glass-ionomer cements bond directly to tooth structures, offer easy handling, possess a coefficient of thermal expansion similar to that of the tooth, and have a potential effect of remineralization. Glass-ionomers are widely used for pedodontic applications and for the restoration of Class III and Class V cavities. They are not recommended for permanent filling of occlusal surfaces in adults where there is excessive load because of insufficient resistance to abrasion.

Metal-reinforced glass ionomers

In the interest of reinforcing glass-ionomer cements, the addition of metals to the filler component has been proposed. The powder contains fluoroaluminosilicate glass and a silver alloy or the glass is sintered with silver. The latter product is called a cermet (ceramic, or glass, and metal). Due to the admixing of metals, these materials are no more tooth colored than other glass-ionomer cements. They have appropriate strength, are easy to manipulate, and are sufficiently radio-opaque. These properties, added to their adhesive ability to the tooth structure make cermet cements appropriate for core buildup. Clinicians may like the difference between the surface hardness of the cement and the tooth structure, and the distinguished color may be helpful when preparing the tooth using burs. Metal-reinforced glass-ionomers also have been proposed as a temporary posterior restorative material[12,13.]

Highly viscous glass-ionomers

Condensable Glass Ionomer cements, more properly termed as High-viscocity GICs,were developed early in the 1990s. The highly viscous glass-ionomer cements were designed as an alternative to amalgam for posterior preventive restorations. These glass-ionomers are particularly useful for the atraumatic restorative treatment (ART) technique. This is a procedure based on excavating carious dentin in teeth using hand instruments only and restoring the tooth with adhesive filling materials. Examples of highly viscous glass-ionomer cements are Fuji IX and Ketac Molar. Such glass-ionomers are expected to be particularly effective in the ART technique when they are applied in the early stages of caries development. According to the manufacturer, the relatively higher viscosity is the result of the addition of poly(acrylic acid) to the powder and finer grain-size distribution. The setting reaction proceeds in accordance with the usual acid-base reaction typical of GICs. Similarly, this group of materials must be differentiated as:

1. Metal-free, eg, Fuji IX, Fuji IX GP, Fuji IX GP Fast, HiFi (Shofu), Ketac-Molar (ESPE).
2. Containing Metal, eg, Hi-Dense (Shofu). Hi-Dense contains metal particles consisting of an alloy of silver, tin, and copper (18 wt%) and titanium oxide (4 wt%).

This class of condensable glass-ionomer cements becomes interesting for primary molar restoration because of the amalgam like properties developed when long mixing times are used. To ensure the constancy of properties, manufactures have sought to provide these products in encapsulated form. A strong macro mechanical preparation without tapered margins should be sought, although some manufacturers suggest increased adhesion to dental hard tissue for this class of material. The minimum layer thickness for these viscous GICs should be approximately 1.5 mm.

The restoration must be covered with a bonding agent immediately after placement to avoid contamination by fluids from the surrounding area. If this is not provided, premature degradation of the restoration is likely. This consideration has led to one manufacturer to offer a low-viscosity monomer especially for use with viscous GIC (Hi-Glaze, Shofu). A second appointment is necessary for final finishing. Despite their relatively fine (by comparison with conventional GIC) particles, these materials are only moderately polishable.

Few definitive studies of viscous GICs are available. Their surface hardness is similar to that of fine-particle hybrid composites. Their abrasion resistance is decisively superior to that of traditional GIC. This is ascribed to other factors, smaller average particle size (Ketac-silver, 14 μm; Ketac-Molar, 2.7 μm) and their related improved distribution within the matrix. Further reduction of the particle size does not seem to lead to less abrasion. An experimental viscous GIC (ESPE) with an average particle size of less than, exhibited significantly higher abrasion than the otherwise compatible Ketac-Molar. Only Viva glass (Ivoclar) is indicated solely for use as a lining material on the basis of its observed tendency to abrade severly and its large particle size. No difference in flexural strength could be established between Hi-Dense, a viscous GIC, and Ketac-Silver, a cermet cement. In general, fluoride release from these materials appears to be similar to that of conventional GIC.

Due to their manipulative and mechanical characteristics, highly viscous glass- ionomers can be used for intermediate restorations, replacing amalgam, and for core buildup procedures. They are applied as glass-ionomer preventive restorations to fill cavities and to seal around them.

Low-viscosity glass ionomers

The low-viscosity glass-ionomers have been developed as liners, fissure protection materials, sealing materials for hypersensitive cervical areas, and endodontic materials. Such materials are designed with low powder-liquid ratios and are highly flowable.

The fluoride released from glass-ionomers strengthens the tooth structure. The low powder: liquid ratio material is expected to cause gradual dissolution from the occlusal surface when they are applied as fissure protection materials. Low-viscosity glass-ionomer cements should be suitable as fissure protection materials during the eruption period of the teeth.

Base and liner

Some glass-ionomers have been developed for base and lining applications. These materials are used for the "sandwich" technique in which they are applied as a dentin substitute and composite resin is applied as an enamel substitute.Thus the advantages of both glass-ionomers and resin composite may be combined. The composite resin shows superior physical and esthetic properties, making it suitable for surface application.

The glass-ionomers show a coefficient of thermal expansion similar to that of the tooth structure, good bonding to dentin, and good biocompatibility, making them suitable for application as a dentin substitute. Some studies also have reported the antibacterial effect of these materials.

Luting

The glass-ionomer cements for luting are widely used for cementing metal inlays, crowns, and bridges. They are considered the most suitable luting cements, because of their ease of manipulation, bonding ability, fluoride release, and low solubility in the oral environment.[21] Their physical properties are well balanced compared to those of zinc phosphate cement, polycarboxylate cement, and resin cement. These cements have gone through many steps in their development. Because the system is complicated, many problems had to be overcome. For example, when comparing the first version of Fuji I for luting and the current product, the physical properties have been improved significantly. As a result, the reliability and durability also have increased.

Resin-Modified Glass-Ionomer Cement

Disadvantages of conventional glass ionomer cements compared to a composite resin are inferior mechanical properties, namely bending strength tensile strength, and fracture toughness.A persisting concern of conventional glass-ionomers is their brittleness and low wear resistance. The latter is even pH-dependent which means that proper oral hygiene is vital[8]. These properties need to be improved in order to widen the range of clinical applications.

For traditional glass-ionomer cement some sort of hybridization at the interaction with the dentin surface has been demonstrated, as is the case with resin bonding and cements, but this form of stable adhesion could be improved for the glass-ionomer cement. Resin modification of glass-ionomer cement was designed to produce favorable physical properties similar to those of resin composites and resin cements while retaining the basic features of the conventional glass-ionomer cement. This goal was achieved by incorporating water-soluble resin monomers into an aqueous solution of polyacrylic acid. In this way the system undergoes polymerization of the resin monomer while the acid-base reaction continues simultaneously. The resulting resin-modified glass-ionomer cements exhibit many advantages of both resin cements and glass-ionomer cements.

The resin-modified glass-ionomer cement is defined as a material that under goes both polymerization reaction and acid-base reaction. The basic composition of the cement liquid is polycarboxylic acid, water, and 2-hydroxyethyl-methacrylate (HEMA). It may also contain a small amount of cross-linking material. Some products, such as Vitremer, are said to contain a polycarboxylic acid modified with pendant methacrylate groups. The composition and structure of the fluoroaluminosilicate glass for resin- modified glass-ionomer cements are basically similar to those of conventional glass-ionomer cements. .

Setting reaction

The essential acid-base reaction between the fluoroaluminosilicate glass and the polycarboxylic acid is initiated by mixing the powder and liquid. At the same time, the polymerization of HEMA and cross- linking material is started by an oxidation- reduction or a photopolymerizing catalyst. This forms a hardened mixture in which HEMA polymer and polycarboxylic acid are supposed to be linked by hydrogen bonding. The acid with polymerizable double bonds that is included in some products is formed with a monomer. Figure.1-11 shows an infrared spectrum illustrating this mechanism in which the resin-modified glass-ionomer cement hardens. The double bonds of the polymerizable monomer included in the liquid disappear after hardening, and the number of carboxyl groups in the polyacrylic acid decreases as the acid- base reaction advances.

One of the main disadvantages of conventional glass-ionomer cement is that when it comes in contact with water during the early stage of setting, the setting reaction is inhibited, damaging the surface of the cement. Water sensitivity could be reduced by incorporating photopolymerization, which promotes faster setting, into the setting reaction.

Rapid setting is also an advantage for color stability. Unlike conventional glass-ionomer cements, after the completion of photo-polymerization hardened resin- modified glass-ionomer cement shows the same shade as a specimen that has been immersed in water for 60 minutes. In other words, water no longer inhibits the setting reaction by the time photo polymerization is completed. The color of the specimen immersed in water soon after photo polymerization is slightly lighter than the control because the resin-modified glass-ionomer cement undergoes both photo and chemical curing, (dual-cured or tricured systems). The chemical setting reaction continues even though the setting reaction initiated by light has been completed. The proportion of chemical setting in the entire process is only about 15%, but this reaction is affected by water. Although the application of varnish is much less effective for reducing water sensitivity in light-cured glass-ionomer cement than in conventional glass-ionomer cement, it is beneficial to prevent contamination from water in resin- modified glass-ionomer cement.

The translucency of resin-modified glass-ionomer cements declines slightly with the lapse of time. The shade of the final restoration is slightly darker than the initial shade, which should be taken into account during shade selection.

During the setting process, the pH of the liquid of resin-modified glass-ionomer cement is about 1.5 because it contains polycarboxylic acid. The pH increases as the acid-base reaction advances. This stage proceeds relatively quickly, probably because the polymerization heat of the monomer promotes the acid-base reaction.

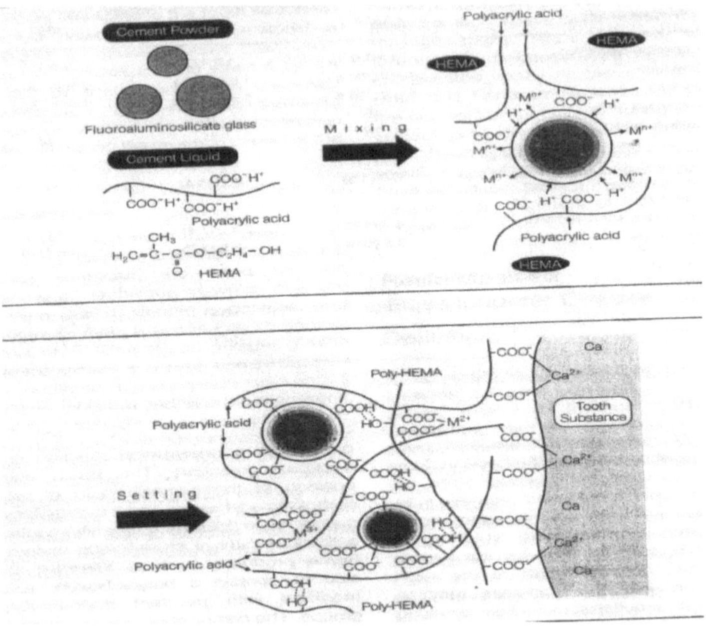

Setting reaction of the resin modified glass ionomer cement.

- H+ ion in the liquid attacks the glass surface
- Metal ion released from the glass particle reacts with polyacrylic acid while HEMA cures concurrently
- Surface layer of glass particle forms a silica gel layer

The setting reaction of RMGIC involves two distinct reactions:

An acid base reaction to hydrolyse the glass and precipitate the coordination and chelation bonded polycarboxylate network and a free radical polymerized network. These network forming reactions have no components in common,even if the functional groups reside on the same physical chain.in either such system alone,reaction increases the viscosity of the mixture,reduces the mobility of the network chain segments,and thus steadily reduces the mobility of the network chain segments,and thus steadily reduces the rate of further reaction until it more or less ceases when the glass transition temperature of the system reaches the ambient tempararture or atleast,the rate drops several orders of magnitude.it is evident from tis that any other processes which may occur and which depend on diffusion are also slowed down as the network forms.Clearly,this must apply to the second network system in combined-chemistry materials.that is th formation processes of the two networks are not kinetically independent,even if chemically distinct.Thus we can make two predictions that if the GI reaction is delayed,the resin network will form more fully but this will then prevent the acid base reaction similarly if the free radical polymerization is delayed the formation of the GI network will proceed unhindered for the time being but this will then prevent the resin network from forming. The first prediction is unstestable as there is no way to switch off the chelating action of the GI polycarboxylate let alone its acidity.however with the light curing system the free radical process can be initiated at will. Furthermore,since the efficiency of the formation of the resin network is the result of a competition between chain formation of the resin network is the result of a competition between chain formation of the resin network is the result network is the result of the a competition between the chain forming and mutual annihilation reactions of the free radicals we can predict an effect due to irradiation time.This must be put in kinetic context :free radical reactions are fast in comparison with the GI reactions,other than the diffusion issues. Thus light activation is expected to result in a rapid initial set thereby reducing sensitivity to moisture,but this means that the GI reaction(which proceeds normally from the point of mixing) is expected to be inhibited once irradiation has occurred.in brief while light curing offers the potential of longer working time this is at the cost of much reduced strength tht cannot be compensated by extra irradiation. There is also an increased risk of leachable resin components that might be toxic. While the generality of these observations needs to be checked by further work the ordinary expectations from the chemistry are presently supported. The rationale for the design and use of these materials must be questioned.

Thus in RMGIC's we can make two predictions:if the GI reaction is delayed,the resin network will form more fully,but this will then prevent the acid base reaction,similarly if the free radical polymerization is delayed,the formation of the GI network will proceed unhindered for the time being but this will then prevent the resin network fro forming.the first prediction is untesteble as there is no way to switch off the chelating action of the GI polycarboxylate,let alone its acidity.However,with a light-curing system the free radical process can be initiated at will.furthermore,since the efficiency of the formation of the resin network is the result of a competition between chain forming and mutual annihilation reactions of the free radicals we can predict an effect due to irradiation time.this must be put in kinetic context:free radical reactions are fast in comparison with the GI reaction,other than the diffusion isuues.it might be imagined that the strengths of rmigic's results from a combination of the strengths of two components.

However it must be noted that this is a combination by replacement not simple addition.The two systems cannot occupy the same space;addition of one means reduction of the other.it is apparent that deviation from the recommended 20s irradiation is associated with lower ollapse stress in marked contrast with filled resin filled resin restorative materials in the case of extra exposure.lower irradiation permits more GI reaction,with its intrinsically weaker structure as shown by the zero irradiation results.more irradiation appears to result in greater free radical mutual annhilation

Adhesion to tooth structures:

It is presumed that the ionic reactivity of a resin-modified glass-ionomer cement to the tooth surface is lower than that of a conventional glass-ionomer cement. However, it can be markedly increased by treating the tooth surface with an acid conditioner. Preparation of the dentin surface with a strong acid such as phosphoric acid weakens the surface's adhesiveness, therefore polyacrylic acid or citric acid are usually used for this purpose. Ferric chloride and aluminum chloride are occasionally used in combination with these acids. It is supposed that these agents stimulate the astringent action of collagen at the interface between the tooth surface and the glass-ionomer cement.

The most notable determinant for how the tooth surface is treated is the use of resin-modified or conventional glass-ionomer cement. Scanning electron micrographs of the cement-enamel and cement-dentin inter- faces with both resin-modified and conventional glass-ionomer cements show that, with conditioning, the resin- modified material apparently forms a hybrid layer whereas the conventional material does not. Treating the enamel surface with phosphoric acid does not decrease the bond of either type of cement, and the bond is stabilized. An aqueous solution of citric acid-ferric chloride or of polyacrylic acid-aluminum chloride also is effective in increasing either cement's adhesiveness. It is probably best to use conditioning materials that exhibit acidity at the same level as that of an aqueous solution of polyacrylic acid and aluminum chloride when both enamel and dentin are treated simultaneously. The bond strength of a resin-modified glass-ionomer cement increases because its tensile strength improves with the treatment. Bond strength was particularly stable after thermal cycling, suggesting the effectiveness of the surface conditioning[21].

Types of resin-modified glass-ionomer cements

Restorative materials

One of the main disadvantages of conventional glass-ionomer cement as a direct restorative material is the need to avoid polishing immediately after placement. This clinical caution is required to prevent deterioration of the material's physical properties caused by water sensitivity during the initial stage of the setting process. The introduction of photo curing to the resin-modified glass-ionomer cement has made the material significantly less sensitive to water.

The popular products in this category are Fuji II LC, Vitremer, and Photac Fil, although their composition and setting mechanisms differ.

Compared with conventional analogs, resin-modified glass-ionomer cements have been characterized as having a longer working time, a rapid set, improved appearance and translucency and higher early strength8,10). these materials is that theycan be finished and polished on the same visit.

The incorporation of monomers and photo polymerization make the material less water-sensitive, while giving it greater mechanical strength and ease of manipulation. It also makes the material more translucent than conventional cements by better matching the refractive indexes of the liquid and the filler. The incorporation of monomers to the cement liquid increases the refractive index of the liquid. In the case of the conventional glass-ionomer Fuji II with a refractive index of 1.42, the liquid of Fuji II LC has a refractive index of 1.44, that brings it nearer to that of the applied glass powder which has a refractive index of 1.50

Base and liner

The first clinical application of resin- modified glass-ionomer cement was as a base and liner. Conventional glass-ionomer products also have been successfully used for these purposes. However, the base and liner applications are usually followed by restorative or temporary filling procedures. Thus, the quick set with photo polymerization of the resin-modified glass-ionomer cement, as opposed to the relatively slow setting of conventional glass-ionomer products, exactly meets the requirements for these applications.

Vitrebond and Fuji Lining LC, products with base and liner applications opened a new era of resin-modified glass-ionomer cements. This type of cement is applied as a liner prior to placement of a composite resin restoration. Fuji Bond LC is a further modification to the lining materials. It was designed to be applied after surface treatment with GC Cavity Conditioner, an aqueous solution of 20% polyacrylic acid with 3% aluminum chloride. The smear layer, which is formed on the cut surface, is removed by a 10-second treatment with the cavity conditioner. The aluminum chloride conditions the dentin surface to enable formation of a hybrid layer with the cement. The powder and liquid of Fuji Bond LC is then thinly mixed with a disposable brush and applied directly to the cavity surface. A thin layer (approximately 10 to 40 μm thick) should be used, allowing the cement to work as both a bonding and a lining material. The monomers penetrate into the demineralized dentin, forming a hybrid layer, which is expected to contribute to long- term stable adhesion of the cement to the tooth. The lining layer of Fuji Bond LC has a low modulus of elasticity and works as a stress relaxation layer, compensating for the stresses developed by the polymerization shrinkage of the composite resin during light curing. Fuji Bond LC also has shown remineralization effects on demineralized cavity walls due to fluoride release.

Resin-modified glass-ionomer cements used as bonding agents prior to placement of composite resins are remarkably different from resin bonding agents. Further development of the former materials are anticipated.

Fissure protection

Conventional glass-ionomer cements for pit and fissure protection offer several advantages. Their ability for long-term fluoride release is beneficial. In addition, glass-ionomers adhere to the tooth structure without acid etching, allowing their use on partially erupted teeth with difficult access for rubber dam isolation. However, although the merits of glass-ionomers used as protection material were accepted in some countries, they were not recognized worldwide. Their retention rate was not as high as that of a resin sealant, and they require prevention of moisture contamination in the early stages of setting. Fuji III LC, a resin- modified glass-ionomer fissure protection material, comprises improved mechanical and handling properties. This material shows a high fluidity and ability to penetrate into fissures. Because the caries morbidity rate is comparatively high for teeth during the eruption period, it is thought that the resin-modified glass-ionomer cement could be an efficient fissure protector. Although this material is retained in the fissure for a required period of time, it does not have to be retained as long as a resin sealant material. Presently, the glass-ionomer cement is the only material that increases the acid resistance of the tooth.

Luting

The bond strength of conventional glass-ionomer cement for luting is not as high as that of resin cement. Failure often occurs as cohesive fractures within the cement. There are many resin-modified glass-ionomers available that contain a monomer component in the liquid to strengthen the matrix of the cured material. Also the bond strength of the material to the tooth structure has been improved with the incorporation of monomers. Fuji Plus and Vitremer luting cements are popular products in this category. They have significantly higher bonding strengths, which has to be attributed to their improved mechanical properties. They undergo the Setting reaction of polymerization by the oxidation-reduction catalyst and conventional acid-base reaction simultaneously. These materials show a sharp setting characteristic in the oral environment, because the polymerization reaction is strongly influenced by environmental temperature, making the material less sensitive to saliva.

Orthodontic cementing material

Significant improvements in its adhesion have made resin-modified glass-ionomer cement applicable as an orthodontic cementing material. Fuji Ortho LC, Fuji Ortho, and Unitek Multi-Cure Glass-ionomer Orthodontic Band Cement have been developed specifically for orthodontic applications. Fuji Ortho is chemically cured and Fuji Ortho LC and Multi-Cure are cured both chemically and by photo polymerization. Although resin cements are the more popular materials for bonding orthodontic brackets because of their reliable bonding strength to both enamel and brackets, they have a major disadvantage. They require acid etching of the substrate prior to bonding procedures. Moreover, the debonding procedure may damage the enamel surface; it has even been reported that the enamel surface of a bonded area was torn off with the bracket during debonding. The treatment of the enamel surface required for bonding with Fuji Ortho LC and Fuji Ortho is conditioning with GC Ortho Conditioner, a 10% aqueous solution of polyacrylic acid. It does not dramatically change the enamel surface like phosphoric acid etching does, but it cleans the surface and promotes a suitable bonding substrate for application of the cement. During orthodontic treatment, the cement release fluoride and prevents demineralization of the enamel around the brackets. The debonding of the brackets is easy and the bonded material can be removed easily with scalers and brush cones. The Unitek Multi-Cure Glass-ionomer Orthodontic Band Cement is specially designed to bond the orthodontic bands. This material sets chemically and also snap-sets with t photo polymerization.

Recenty a new anhydrous GIC for bonding of orthodontic brackets was introduced,orthocem B(PSP dental Co,LTD U.K)no acid etching is required for this cement.

In a review of literature by Sidhu.K.S where the clinical evaluations of RMGIC's was done under the headings of retention,marginal characteristics,material deterioration,secondary caries,color stability as well as pu lpal and biological effects. The clinical observations were done over a period of 13years by different researchers and they concluded that RMGIC'swell in terms of retention,secondary caries as well as post operative sensitivity and results were little compromising in terms of marginal characteristics,surface properties and color stability[24].

Polyacid-Modified Resin Composites

In the search for a new restoration material, an attempt was made to polymerize an acid monomer in the presence of fluoroaluminosilicate glass. This attempt led to the development of a compound that releases fluoride slowly in the oral environment; it is called compomer. The compomer shows physical properties quite similar to those of composite resin. At the same time, the acid monomer which has been polymerized exhibits acidity when in contact with water from the saliva and reacts with the basic glass which contains fluoride.

Two types of material exist between the extremes represented by composite resins and conventional glass-ionomer cements: resin-modified glass-ionomer cements and compomers. The nature and physical properties of these materials can be modified consecutively between the two extremes. Therefore, several products claim to have the nature of both conventional glass-ionomer cements and composite resin, making the classification of such materials complicated. The compomer is one of the materials in this category. It basically has a similar nature and similar physical properties to resin composites. According to the manufacturers, it also has the ability to release fluoride and undergoes an acid-base reaction between the acidic monomer and basic glass filler in the presence of water in the saliva. However, the compomer does not contain water and does not self-adhere to the tooth structure, which distinguishes it from a resin-modified glass-ionomer material. The compomer is mainly a resin composite with fiuoride-releasing potential.

Basic composition

The compomer is a one-paste material consisting of fillers and a matrix that is similar to that of composite resin. Each compomer product has a different composition of fillers and matrix, depending on the manufacturer's technology. The material usually contains fluoroaluminosilicate glass powder as filler to release fluoride. Metal fluoride also is included in some materials for the same purpose. The fluoroaluminosilicate glass contains strontium or some other metal to make the material radiopaque. The compomer's original composition contained the acidic monomer in its matrix, although the other part of the matrix is similar to that of composite resin.

The polymerization reaction of the monomer components, initiated by photo polymerization rules the setting reaction of the compomer. The acidic monomer is polymerized with other monomer components of the matrix to the acidic polymer, or the polymer with acidic group, in the initial setting reaction. The acid- base reaction is inhibited until the material hardens and absorbs water. The material is said to have its acid-base reaction between the acid group in the polymer and the basic glass filler in the presence of water from the saliva.

Clinical application of compomers

Some of the compomers available are Dyract AP, Compoglass F, F2OOO, and lonosit Fil. These products are light-cured, one-paste materials that are capable of fluoride release. The main clinical application for compomers is restorative filling, because they are not adhesive and require a separate bonding agent. Compomers possess better mechanical properties and manipulability than glass-ionomer filling materials, and their flowability in the cavity is better than that of resin composite. However, the need for application of a bonding agent prior to filling is a disadvantage, and the mechanical properties of compomers are inferior to those of resin composites. Presently, the compomer can be classified as an intermediate material between the glass ionomer for filling and the resin composite. Long-term clinical studies with the compomers are expected, in which the clinical benefits to patients will be identified clearly.

5. RECENT MODIFICATIONS OF GIC

Smart Materials:

It was traditional in the older literature to identify dental materials as those materials essentially or desirably inert in the mouth. This definition is longer valid – as shown by fluoride-containing materials, which are by definition not inert because they release fluoride ions.

The development of fluoride-releasing materials faces two problems :

1. The more effective the fluoride release, the more open is the structure of the material : this is often associated with low strength.
2. As fluoride-containing materials are made more dense and strong, the efficiency of ion release is reduced. This is usually characterized by a burst of fluoride release followed by a rapid decline in the ion release rate. Essentially in such cases the fluoride is emanating only from the superficial layer of the material.
   Two approaches have been suggested to improve the therapeutic potenetial of fluoride-releasing materials, both of which may produce materials that are therapeutically active and mechanically strong.

'Fluoride Charge' Materials

A fluoride charge material is a modified glass ionomer, and is a two-part material.The restorative part of the material is used in the same way, typically in paedodontic cases. When the first burst of the fluoride is expended and the therapeutical potential of the restoration is spent, the material can be given a second fluoride 'charge' using a gel material that replenishes the fluoride sites in the restorative by ion exchange and recovers the fluoride release and therapeutic potential of restorative. This ofcourse is achived without the need to replace the material, provided the restoration meets the normal standards of anatomical sufficiency.

This approach is still at the experimental stage and several workers are evaluating the approach.

Low pH

A second approach to optimize fluoride materials takes account of the fact that : Fluoride release may be most beneficial at low pH, when caries attack may be most threatening. This has given rise to materials that may be properly called 'smart' because they use a low oral pH to increase fluoride release. The fluoride is thus not released all the time; this episodic release prolongs the therapeutic usefulness of the material and optimizes the fluoride release.

Bioactive Glass

The idea of a bioactive glass was developed by Hench and co-workers in 1973. Dissolution of the glass stimulates the formation of a layer rich in calcium phosphate, which can bond to bone. The applications of this in various types of bone augmentation, including the atropic lower mandible, are obvious. Use of bioactive glasses has also been suggested for the correction of infra-bony pockets in periodontology.

However, the use of bioactive glasses may have a greater application in the ceramic restorations for the crown of the teeth. When the formulation is a bioglass-ceramic, strength may be further improved. Bioactive glass may have a number of other advantages.

As already noted, bioactive glasses 'grow' calcium phosphate rich layers in the presence of calcium and phosphate saturated saliva. These may repair surface flaws, which are widely beliced to be responsible for the low strength of ceramics

Bioactive glasses can be formulated that are much less abrasive than feldspathic porcelain, and thus less aggressive on the enamel of opposing teeth. Trauma to the opposing enamel is one of the most important contraindications to the use of dental porcelain, especially in bruxists and in cases where larger area of porcelain are involved.

In the university of Minnesota, Francis et al are persuing the possibility that bioacyive glasses may also be made to bind to dentin. In the best of cases one can envisage a bioactive porcelain jacket crown withgreater longevity, less trauma to the dentition and with inherent adhesive properties to dentin. Such crowns could be contoured with thinner facial cross section, giving better angle of emergence without loss of strength. Further, processing temperatures would be lower than those currently used for more conventional ceramics.

These materials are also in their infancy, and even if the chemical problems can be solved, there remains the problem of anterior esthetics. This might mean that the first candidate bioactive porcelain jacket crowns would be consigned to posterior teeth.

Glass Ionomers: Bio Active Implant Materials

Glass-ionomer cements (GICs) originally designed for use as dental materials have a number of advantages over acrylic bone cements. These include lack of exotherm during setting, absence of monomer and improved release of incorporated therapeutic agents; this has resulted in the development of GICs for biomedical applications. Major landmarks in this history are the formulation of defined-composition ionomer glasses and an improved understanding of the biological and material properties of GICs. Following implantation, GICs can form a stable integration with bone, and affect the growth and development of bone, both adjacent to their surface and systemically, through an ion release mechanism. The 'non-inert' nature of this group of materials is also demonstrated by their adverse effects on neural tissue. Successful clinical use of GICs, both as bone cements and as preformed implants for hard tissue replacement, have been reported in the fields of otologic surgery (Cochlear implant fixation, repair of the tympanic chain, eustation tube obliteration and as ear ossicles), and oral and reconstructive surgery. If the material is to be used to bridge ossicular chain defects, anchor cochlear implants and stabilize ossicular reconstruction prosthesis,it must be capable of maintaining a bond between these materials and structures and a study was designed to answer the following questions. Will bacteria in vitro adhere to the cement?Will bacteria in vitro affect the cement? Do different pH levels affect the cement? Significant amounts of calcium, and presumably other components, are released into solution from the cement at all pH levels.Exposure to bacteria in vitro accelerates loss of matrix on the prosthesis surface and bacteria readily adhere to the cement surface. Until further study is conducted, use of the cement in contact with cerebral spinal fluid should be avoided.The use of GICs in situations where they will come into contact with nerves or neural tissue is contraindicated.

Experimental studies on a new bioactive material: HAIonomer cements.

The lack of exotherm during setting, absence of monomer and improved release of incorporated therapeutic agents has resulted in the development of glass ionomer cements (GICs) for biomedical applications. In order to improve biocompatibility and biomechanically match GICs to bone, hydroxyapatite-ionomer (HAIonomer) hybrid cements were developed. Ultra-fine hydroxyapatite (HA) powders were produced using a new induction spraying technique that utilizes a radio-frequency source to spheriodize an atomized suspension containing HA crystallites. The spheriodized particulates were then held at 800 degrees C for 4 h in a carbolite furnace using a heating and cooling rate of 25 degrees C/min to obtain almost fully crystalline HA powders. The heat-treated particles were characterized and introduced into a commercial glass ionomer cement. 4 (H4), 12 (H12) and 28 (H28) vol% of fluoroalumino silicate were substituted by crystalline HA particles that were dispersed using a high-speed dispersion technique. The HAIonomer cements were subjected to hardness, compressive and diametral tensile strength testing based upon BS6039:1981. The storage time were extended to one week to investigate the effects of cement maturation on mechanical properties. Commercially available capsulated GIC (GC) and GIC at maximum powder:liquid ratio (GM) served as comparisons. Results were analyzed using factorial ANOVA/Scheffe's post-hoc tests and independent samples t-test at significance level 0.05. The effect of time on hardness was material dependent. With the exception of H12, a significant increase in hardness was observed for all materials at one week. A significant increase in compressive strength was, however, observed for H12 over time. At 1 day and 1 week, the hardness of H28 was significantly lower than for GM, H4, and H12. No significant difference in compression and diametral tensile strengths were observed between materials at both time intervals. Results show that HAIonomers is a promising material, which possess good mechanical properties. Potential uses of this new material include bone cements and performed implants for hard tissue replacement in the field of otological, oral-maxillofacial and orthopedic surgery.

Structure of bioactive glass and its application to glass ionomer cement.

A new glass ionomer cement was prepared, using bioactive CaO-P2O5-SiO2(MgO) glass and setting process was investigated using FT-IR and MAS NMR analyses. The compressive strengths of the cements depended on the glass composition and a maximum strength of 33.3 +/- 4.7 MPa was obtained using cement with the glass composition of MgO:4.6, CaO:44.9, SiO2:34.2 and P2O5:16.3% in weight. FT-IR analysis showed that the COOH group in the polyacrylic acid decreased and carboxylate ion (COO-Ca2+) increased after the setting reaction. A broad signal appeared around -82 ppm in 29Si MAS-NMR spectra of the glass and a new signal corresponding to hydrated silica gel formation appeared around -102 and -111 ppm after setting. This suggests that Ca2+ was released from the glass powder to form carboxylate salt and that a degree of polymerization in the silicate network increased. The setting mechanism of the cement was found to be essentially the same as in conventional glass ionomer cement.

Effect of polyacrylic acid on the apatite formation of a bioactive ceramic in a simulated body fluid: fundamental examination of the possibility of obtaining bioactive glass-ionomer cements for orthopaedic use.

Glass-ionomer cements, which consist of CaO-Al2O3-SiO2-CaF2 glass powders and a polyalkenoic acid solution, such as polyacrylic acid (PAA), have been widely used in dentistry. They set rapidly without any shrinkage, the lack of temperature increase on reaction, and develop high mechanical strength. Therefore, if bioactive glass-ionomer cements can be obtained, such cements are expected to be useful as cements for fixing orthopaedic implants to the surrounding bone. In the present study, to examine the possibility of obtaining bioactive glass-ionomer cements, the effect of PAA on the apatite formation on bioactive ceramics in a simulated body fluid was investigated. It was revealed that presence of even a small quantity of PAA inhibits the apatite formation in the body environment. It is speculated that when glass-ionomer cements are implanted into the body, PAA can be released from the glass-ionomer cements and inhibits the apatite formation on their surfaces. It is reasonable to suppose that this will occur with any glass-ionomer cement that contains PAA. Therefore, it might be considered difficult to obtain bioactive glass-ionomer cements.

Compound changes and tooth mineralization effects of glass ionomer cements containingbioactiveglass(S53P4).

Modifications of glass ionomer cements (GICs) were made by adding bioactive glass (BAG) to GIC to obtain bioactive restorative materials. This study used SEM, EDS and visual analysis to examine the bioactivity and the ability of the study materials to mineralize dentin. Conventional cure and resin-modified light-curing GIC were used. The materials consisted of powder and liquid. Three experimental materials were made by mixing 10-30 wt% of BAG powder with GIC powders. Commercially available GIC without BAG were used as controls. Class III restorations were made in altogether 62 intact beagle dog teeth, and the operation was performed under general anesthesia. The restorations were followed clinically for 1, 3 or 6 weeks. Resin-modified GIC containing BAG showed uniform CaP surface formation on the restorations. Mineral depositions in the close vicinity of the restoration-dentin interface and in deeper parts of dentin tubules were also noticed in resin-modified GIC containing BAG particles. It can be concluded that resin-modified GIC containing BAG have good potential in clinical applications where enhanced mineralization is expected.

Release of silica, calcium, phosphorus, and fluoride from glass ionomer cement containing bioactive glass.

The aim of this study was to examine the release of silica (Si), calcium (Ca), phosphorous (P), and fluoride (F) from conventional glass ionomer cement (GI) and resin-modified glass ionomer cement (LCGI), containing different quantities of bioactive glass (BAG). Further aim was to evaluate in vitro biomineralization of dentine. The release of Si increased with the increasing immersion time from the specimens containing BAG, whereas the amount of Ca and P decreased indicating in vitro bioactivity of the materials. LCGI with 30wt% of BAG showed highest bioactivity. It also showed CaP-like precipitation on both the surface of the test specimens and on the dentin discs immersed with the material. Within the limitations of this study, it can be concluded that a dental restorative material consisting of glass ionomer cements and BAG is bioactive and initiates biomineralization on dentin surface in vitro.

GIOMERS :

Giomers are a relatively new type of restorative material. The name "giomer" is a hybrid of the words "glass ionomer" and "composite", which pretty well describes what a giomer is claimed to be. Although glass-ionomer restorative materials such as Ketac-Fil (3M ESPE) and Fuji Type II (GC America) have some very important properties, such as fluoride release, fluoride rechargeability, and chemical bonding to tooth structure, they also have well-known shortcomings. Their esthetics, for example, are less than ideal and make them a poor second choice to resin composites for restoring esthetically-demanding areas. Also, they are sensitive to moisture contamination and desiccation, which can present the clinician with challenges during their placement. In the 1990s manufacturers improved these shortcomings by adding resins to glass ionomers to produce resin-modified glass ionomers. These products (e.g., Fuji II LC, GC America; Vitremer, 3M ESPE; Photac-Fil Quick, 3M ESPE) have much better esthetics and handling characteristics than glass ionomers. Importantly, they also retain many of the glass ionomer's beneficial properties, such as long-term fluoride release and the ability to be recharged with topically-applied fluoride. They tend, however, to discolor over time. In another attempt to "better" the glass ionomer restorative materials, compomers were also developed. They were touted as being similar to glass ionomers but having much better esthetics and being easier to place and polish. Unfortunately, some of the manufacturer's claims were not confirmed by published research. Although they handled better than GICs, they released much less fluoride and could not be recharged.

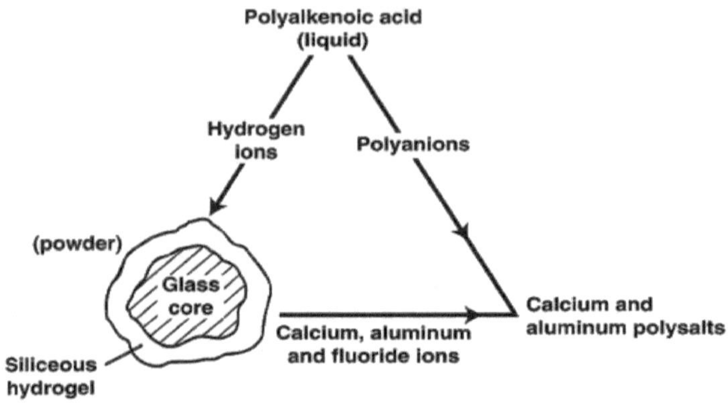

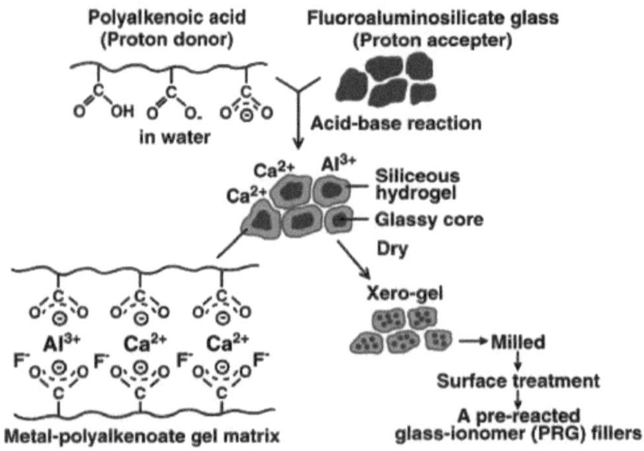

In the continuing quest for improved glass ionomer-like restoratives, manufacturers have developed and introduced a new class of materials called "giomers." As noted earlier, the term implies they are combinations of glass ionomers and composites. Their manufacturers claim they have properties of both glass ionomers (fluoride release, fluoride recharge) and resin composites

(excellent esthetics, easy polishability, biocompatibility). Robertset *al.*17) remarked the fact that the fluoride-releasing mechanism of glass-ionomer cement was derived from its acid-base reaction phase, and invented a revolutionary PRG filler technology. PRG fillers were fabricated by the acid-base reaction between fluoride containing glass (such as FASG) and polyacrylic acid(such as PAA) in the presence of water to form a wet siliceous hydrogel. After freeze-drying, the desiccated xerogel was further milled and silanized to form PRG fillers of a specific size range Giomers are distinguished by the fact that, while they are resin-based, they contain pre-reacted glass-ionomer (PRG) particles. The particles are made of fluorosilicate glass that has been reacted with polyacrylic acid prior to being incorporated into the resin. The pre-reaction can involve only the surface of the glass particles (called surface pre-reacted glass ionomer or S-PRG) or almost the entire particle (termed fully pre-reacted glass ionomer or F-PRG). Optimal filler content has been identified as 17 wt% PRG fillers in adhesive, as the product showed strong adhesion to enamel and dentin with a favorable amount of fluoride release. Dynamic SIMS analysis indicated that fluoride released from the PRG fillers in the adhesive penetrated the dentin substrate though the bonding interface[30].
TEM images of the PRG-Ca fillers showed that dehydrated hydrogels were barely distinguishable from normal glass fillers, if not for the concurrent presence of remnant, incompletely reacted glass cores. On bonding durability, it was found that the improved durability of resin-dentin bonds might be achieved not only *via* the strengthened dentin due to fluoride ion uptake from the PRG-Ca fillers, but also due to retention of relatively insoluble 4-AETCa formed around remnant apatite crystallites within the hybrid layer in 4-AET-containing self-etching adhesives. Further, it was expected that uptake of fluoride ions with cariostatic effect from PRG-Ca fillers would endow dentin substrates with the benefit of secondary caries prevention, together with an effective and durable adhesion to dentin. To leverage on the newly developed PRG filler technology and toreap the multiple benefits rendered by PRG fillers, Shofu Inc. has proposed a new category coined as"Giomer" (Glass ionomer + polymer). To date, 10 kinds of fluoride-releasing "Giomer products" have been developed.[28]

Only one giomer is commercially available presently, ***Shofu's Beautiful***, which uses the S-PRG technology. According to Shofu, Beautiful is indicated for restoring Class I through V lesions as well as for treating cervical erosion lesions and root caries. It is available in 13 shades and is supplied in syringes.

Little published research is available on the properties or performance of giomers. One recently published study compared the fluoride release of a glass ionomer, a resin-modified glass ionomer, a giomer, and a compomer. It found that while the giomer released fluoride, it did not have an initial "burst" type of release like glass ionomers, and its long-term (i.e., 28-day) release was lower than that of the other materials. Another study found that a giomer, after polishing with Sof-Lex disks, had a smoother surface than a glass ionomer, and one that was comparable to that of a compomer and a resin composite. A three-year clinical study comparing the performance of a giomer with that of a microfill resin composite in Class V erosion/abrasion/abfraction lesions has also been done. After measuring eight performance characteristics, no significant differences between the two materials were found.

Chlorhexidine Containing Glass Ionomer Cement:

Glass ionomer cement with addition of chlorhexidine used as a varnish on tooth surfaces has been shown to reduce the number of interproximal mutans streptococci (ms). The effect of a single application of such a varnish containing 2.5% chlorhexidine on occlusal caries development of the first permanent molars on 6-year-old children in a high caries incidence area was investigated. The children were examined according to WHO criteria and 262 children with 2 caries free contra-lateral molars were selected for treatment. Salivary ms samples were collected using the Strip-mutans (SM) method. After brushing the occlusal surfaces with a toothbrush and pumice in water slurry, rinsing and drying with a cotton roll, glass ionomer cement containing chlorhexidine (GI-CHX) and glass ionomer (GI) were applied randomly with a micro brush and the varnish was covered with occlusal wax. At baseline, the mean defs was 18.18 and DMFS was 0.25 and after one year 18.24 and 0.83 respectively. The salivary ms scores were high or very high (SM 2 and 3) in 85.6% at baseline. At the one-year follow up, the GI-CHX and GI materials could not be detected in the fissures. Also, a large number of fissure sealants had been placed in the molars outside the study protocol; thus 4% of the GI-CHX and GI, and 70% of the untreated were sealed at year one. Overall, there was no significant difference between the caries-reducing effect of GI-CHX and GI, but a trend towards a higher effect was seen for GI-CHX. Excluding the sealed molars the reduction was 74% in the GI-CHX-group, and 71% in the GI-group. Conclusion: Addition of 2.5% chlorhexidine to glass ionomer did not seem to increase the caries-reducing effect of the varnish in this high caries incidence population.

Resin modified glass-ionomers combined with chlorhexidine.

A study was conducted to determine the effect on mechanical properties and antimicrobial activity of the addition of chlorhexidine (CHX) to a resin modified glass-ionomer (Photac-fil, ESPE, Norristown, PA, USA). Chlorhexidine diacetate was combined with a resin modified glass-ionomer material at a concentration of 5%. The samples were tested for hardness, tensile strength and erosion at 24 h and 6-week intervals and for elution of CHX and antimicrobial activity weekly for 6 weeks. At 24 h there was no significant difference in hardness between the two groups, but at 6 weeks the resin modified glass-ionomer group was significantly harder than the CHX groups ($P < 0.05$). The diametral tensile strength test indicated no difference between the control and CHX groups at 24 h or at 6 weeks. The jet erosion test demonstrated significantly less erosion with the CHX group at 24 h but at 6 weeks the CHX group showed significantly more erosion than the control group. The chemical assay data demonstrated a peak elution of CHX at week 1 with residual amounts at weeks 2 and 3. The microbial data demonstrated that the CHX group had a significant reduction in Streptococcus mutans numbers for weeks 1-3, but after week 4 there was no difference between the glass-ionomer with and without CHX. The addition of CHX to resin modified glass-ionomer altered hardness and erosion of the resin-modified glass-ionomer, but because there are no material specifications, it is difficult to determine clinical implications. Chlorhexidine did significantly improve the antimicrobial effect of the glass-ionomer which was consistent with the chemical assay data. The results indicated that the addition of CHX to resin modified glass-ionomer material (Photac-fil) did not seriously degrade the physical properties during the time period tested and that the addition of CHX resulted in a greater reduction in S. mutans when compared with glass-ionomer alone.

6. SETTING REACTION

The Setting Reaction and its Clinical Consequences :

The setting characteristics of the glass ionomer cement are central to its science, and some understanding of the setting reaction-even if only in outline-is needed to appreciate the scientific technology of glass-ionomer cements and the correct clinical usage of them in dental surgery.

Poor setting behaviour was the drawback of early glass-ionomer cements, because the clinical consequences of progressive setting are not confined to premature loss of workability and sluggish hardening but extend to other properties. Set cements that are not fully hardening prolongs this period of sensitivity. Thus, the clinician must devote much attention to keeping the restoration protected from saliva.

The vulnerability of the freshly set cement to water can be best appreciated by considering the chemistry of the setting reaction. Fortunately, although the setting reaction is extremely complex and is imperfectly understood in detail and it is doubtful if the reaction will ever be fully unraveled-the outline of the reaction is simple to describe and understand.

Chemistry of the setting :

When the cement powder and aqueous liquid are brought together to form a paste, the glass powder, which is basic, reacts with the poly (alkenoic acid), often poly (acrylic acid), to form a salt hydrogel. This hydrogel is the binding matrix. Water is the reaction medium and is also an essential part of the hydrogel, for it is required to hydrate the metal polyalkenoate formed.

The glass-ionomer cement sets and hardens by a transfer of metal ions from the glass to the poly(acrylic acid), which causes gelation in the aqueous phase. During the process of transfer the matrix-forming metal ions are in soluble form and vulnerable to attack by aqueous fluids. Some form of limited protection during this period is essential.

There is another reason for protection. Water forms an important part of the cement structure, and loss of water of hydration disrupts the cement structure. Loss of water can occur before the cement has fully matured, for example by dehydration or vigorous finishing techniques. Once the cement has fully matured-and this may take many days – this is no longer a problem.

The chemistry of the cement-forming reaction from initial mixing through the various stages of the reaction is depicted.

1) ***Decomposition*** of the glass and release of cement-forming metal ions (Al^{3+} and Ca^{2+}).
2) ***Migration*** of these metal ions into the aqueous phase of the cement.
3) ***Gelation*** of the polyacid by the metal ions leading to set.

4) ***Post-set hardening*** when metal ions become increasingly bound to the polyacid chain. Under conditions of high humidity, the cement tends to expand. The cement is vulnerable to moisture until sufficient hardness has developed. This can take up to one hour but is generally less for modern materials. Hardening continues for about 24 hours, during which time translucency develops as the chemical reaction proceeds.
5) ***Further slow maturation.*** Even after 24 hours a further slow maturation takes place and in the first few days translucency develops further, as does resistance to desiccation and acid attack. Over a period of months the cement becomes more rigid and gathers strength. The reaction is slightly exothermic, the exotherm being less than that of any of the other water-based cements. This exotherm is reflected in a setting shrinkage, however, which can be nullified by hydroscopic expansion.

A full account of the setting reactions, as much as it is known, is given below. It is based largely on the work of Crisp and Wilson (1974a, 1974b), Crisp et al. (1974), Crisp and Wilson (1976), Wilson et al, (1976), Prosser et al. (1982b), and Cook (1983). Most of their work was carried out using the glass G-200 and poly(acrylic acid). Although now other glasses and other polyacids are also used in glass-ionomer cements, the results of these studies can generally be applied to them all.

Decomposition of the glass and migration of ions:

In the early stages of the reaction, the glass powder is decomposed by the polyacid a property characteristic of this type of glass (Crisp and Wilson, 1974a). In a normal cement mix where there is a considerable excess of powder over liquid, about 20% to 30% of the glass is attacked. The attack occurs at the surface of the glass, and as cations are withdrawn the glass network breaks down into silicic acid, which polymerizes at the surface of the glass powder. Ions locked up in the glass network-principally Al^{3+}, Ca^{2+}, and F^- - are released and migrate into the aqueous phase of the cement, the aluminium and fluoride as complexes. Calcium ions predominate because the acid attack on the glass is not uniform, but occurs preferentially at calcium-rich sites (Barry et al., 1979).

As the reaction proceeds the concentration of these ions increases, with the preferential buildup of calcium over aluminium. The pH also increases, which reflects the conversion of the poly(acrylic acid) to polyacrylates. The viscosity of the paste also increases as the poly(acrylic acid), originally in a random coil configuration, acquires charge and unwinds under the influence of electrostatic forces of repulsion. {of metal ions}

Gelation and vulnerability to water :

At a critical pH and ionic concentration precipitation of insoluble polyacrylates begins to take place. When this process reaches a certain stage, the cement sets. Even after set, in the post set hardening phase, the precipitation process continues–indeed, it is responsible for the development of hardness – until all the ions are in insoluble form.

The studies of Crisp et al. (1974) and Barry et al. (1979) have shown that calcium polyacrylate is responsible for the initial set at least in the absence of tartrate, but that the hardening process derives from the slower formation of aluminium polyacrylate, which phase ultimately predominates in the matrix.

Not all the carboxyl (COOH) groups of poly(acrylic acid) are converted to carboxylate groups (COO^-) during the course of the reaction, for two reasons. First, when most of the carboxylic acid groups have ionized, the negative charge on the polymer chain has increased to such an extent that the positively charged hydrogen ions become very strongly bound to the remaining un-ionized carboxylic acid groups and are not easily replaced by metal ions. Second, as the density of cross-links increases the metal ions are increasingly hindered in their movements toward carboxyl sites.

What is important for the clinician to remember is that after set, but before the cement is fully hardened, a proportion of the cement-forming aluminium, calcium, fluoride, and polyacrylate ions are in soluble form and so can be dissolved out of the cement by aqueous fluids. Once these ions are leached out they are irretrievably lost for matrix formation and the cement is permanently weakened. In particular, the surface is softened and becomes opaque as water is absorbed, causing the restoration to lose its aesthetic appeal (Mount and Makinson, 1982).

Ions released from the glass accumulate in the cement water and subsequently are removed by precipitation. The concentration of soluble ions reaches a maximum as the glass is decomposed, and then declines as the insoluble matrix is formed. The object of a manufacturer developing the cement is to reduce this period of vulnerability to a minimum by sharpening the rate of hardening.

Although glass-ionomer cements have been improved considerably, for the best clinical results it is still advisable to adopt a strict routine to exclude water during this vulnerable stage of setting.

In this connection, calcium polyacrylate, which is more vulnerable to water than aluminium polyacrylate, is believed to predominate in freshly set cements–further reason for protecting the freshly set cement. Indeed, one manufacturer has attempted to improve his product by washing the glass powder with acid to remove calcium ions from the surface (Schmidt et al., 1981). This process delays initial set and gives excellent working and setting characteristics.

Causes of gelation :

So far we have explained why calcium and aluminium ions, simple or complex, cause the polyacrylate to gel. Sodium ions do not have this effect and it is tempting to conclude that the divalent calcium and trivalent aluminium ions cross-link the polyacrylate chains ionically.

The coordination of the aluminium ion has to be considered. The coordination number of aluminium is six in the presence of water; that is, there must be six ligands attached to a central aluminium ion. The ligands in the case of glass-ionomer cements would be COO^- from polyacrylate, F^- ions, OH^- ions, and water molecules. However, it is easy to see how the $\{AlF.3H_2O)^{2+}$ unit can bridge just two polyacrylate chains.

However, gelation may simply be caused by the multivalent aluminium and calcium ions displacing or partly displacing the various spheres of hydration that interpose themselves between the cation-anion ion pairs. Contact cation-polyacrylate ion pairs are formed; the cations are site-bound. Desolvation of hydration spheres renders the ionic pairs more hydrophobic and precipitation occurs. Sodium ions cannot displace the hydration sphere and are not site bound because of their low ionic charge. Consequently, they do not precipitate as polyacrylates.

In this model, cross-linking does not play a dominant role, the cohesive binding forces in the cement being attributable, in the main, to chain entanglement. Recent experimental evidence (Hill et al., 1986) indicates that chain entanglement, weak ionic cross-linking, and hydrogen bonds are all involved in matrix formation.

Hardening and slow maturation :

Hardening and the precipitation process continue for about 24 hours and are accompanied by a slight expansion under conditions of high humidity and the development of translucency. Further changes continue to take place for a considerable period – at least a year and probably more.

There are a number of indicators of these slow changes. In the first few days the translucency of the cement improves and the cement becomes resistant to desiccation. Strength continues to increase for at least a year and is apparently proportional to the logarithm of time. The cement, which initially shows some plastic character, like the zinc polycarboxylate cement, becomes increasingly rigid as it ages until it approaches the rigidity of the phosphate-bonded cements (Paddon and Wilson, 1976). This behaviour is unique among the dental cements. Also, the ability of the cement to absorb or lose water decreases as it ages.

The underlying chemical changes causing these physical changes remain a subject for debate. But Wilson and his coworkers have shown that increases in strength are associated with increases in bound water ; that is, increasing hydration of the metal-carboxylate links in a manner analogous to the hydration reactions in Portland cement (Wilson et al., 1979 ; Wilson et al., 1981). This progressive hydration explains the increasing stability of the cement with regard to gain or loss of water.

Increasing strength and rigidity must be associated with a slow increase in cross-linking. There is some evidence for such a time-dependent increase in cross-linking, for it has recently been observed that the glass transition temperature of the cement rises with time (Hill, 1986). Increase in cross-linking could result from slow replacement of residue carboxyl hydrogen predominance of aluminium over calcium in the matrix.

Cement structure :

Knowledge of the structure of glass-ionomer cement comes from studies by : Barry et al. (1979) and Brune and Smith (1982). The set cement is a highly complex composite, where a cored filler is bound together by a hydrogel of calcium and aluminium polyacrylates that contains fluorine, probably as a fluoroaluminium polyacrylate.

The filler system is complex and is derived from the original glass powder, which is partly degraded to a siliceous hydrogel that apparently contains fluorite crystallites. The larger filler particles contain a glassy core pitted by selective etching and sheathed by a siliceous hydrogel. Observation indicates that the bond between core and sheath is not particularly strong. The smaller filler particles are composed entirely of a siliceous hydrogel that can be presumed to be completely degraded relics of small glass particles.

The nature of the cohesive forces binding the matrix together is a subject for speculation, but they can be presumed to be a mixture of ionic cross-links, hydrogen bridges, and chain entanglements.

The role of water

The glass-ionomer cements are water-based materials, and water plays an important role in their setting and structure. It is the reaction medium into which the cement-forming cations- calcium and aluminium- are leached and in which they are transported to react with the polyacid to form a polyacrylate matrix. Water also serves to hydrate the siliceous hydrogel and the metal polyacrylate salts formed. It is an essential part of the cement structure. If water is lost from the cement by desiccation while it is setting, the cement-forming reactions will stop.

Water present in the set cement can be classified, somewhat arbitrarily, into two forms: "loosely bound" water, which is readily removed by desiccation, and "tightly bound" water, which cannot be removed (Wilson and Crisp, 1975 ; Crisp et al., 1976c ; Elliott et al., 1975 ; Wilson et al., 1979 ; Wilson et al., 1981). Tightly bound water is associated with the hydration shell of the cation-polyacrylate bond, particularly that of aluminium, and some silica gel water.

As the cement ages, the degree of hydration, that is, the ratio of tightly bound to loosely bound water, increases. This is accompanied by an increase in strength and modulus and a decrease in plasticity (Paddon and Wilson, 1976 ; Wilson et al., 1981).

Water is easily lost and gained by the cement, as the loosely bound water is labile ; indeed, the cement is only stable in an atmosphere of 80% relative humidity (Hornsby, 1980). In higher humidities, the cement absorbs water and the consequent hydroscopic expansion can exceed the setting shrinkage. This is a clinical advantage. The cement can lose water under drying conditions, however, leading to shrinking and crazing. The earliest clinical observations of this phenomenon were made by J.W. McLean with ASPA I in the early 1970s. Moreover, loss of water will retard cement formation, since it is the reaction medium, and will prevent strength from fully developing, since it is required for the hydration of the matrix salts.

Susceptibility to desiccation decreases as the cement ages (Saito, 1978 ; Hornsby, 1980). The period of vulnerability is different for different cements and has been stated to range from one to 30 days depending on the material used (Phillips and Bishop, 1985). Paradoxically early contact with moisture is equally damaging. Glass-ionomer cements rapidly absorb water, mainly in the first day (Crisp et al., 1976c, 1980). If the cement is not sufficiently mature, this can lead to disruption of the surface by swelling or loss of substance to the oral environment, which results in surface roughness (Wilson et al., 1981 ; Causton, 1981 ; Roulet and Walti, 1984 ; Philips and Bishop, 1985). However, if glass-ionomer cements are protected for between ten and 30 minute, depending on brand, this problem does not arise.

Thus, glass-ionomer cements must be protected against two extremes: desiccation and aqueous fluids. It is a question of water balance, and as we have seen this is achieved in an atmosphere of 80% relative humidity. Higher humidities are not harmful, for the cement will then absorb water and expand. But contact with aqueous fluids must be avoided, for these remove, irretrievably, cement-forming ions

Protection :

What are the clinical implications of this need for water balance ?

A rubber dam, while useful in protecting the unset cement from moisture, can have a damaging effect by allowing the cement paste to desiccate. Desiccation will retard the reaction, and can cause shrinking and crazing once the cement has set. At this stage of the clinical procedure, the clinician should work with the cement exposed to the humid condition of the mouth while at the same time ensuring that moisture droplets do not contaminate the surface of the cement.

Once set, and after the matrix has been removed, the cement should be protected by a suitable barrier. The period of protection against moisture can be quite short. Sixty minutes will usually suffice, but the exact period depends on the brand used (Mount and Makinson, 1982; Phillipsand Bishop, 1985).

As yet there appears to be no ideal barrier for the purpose (Earl et al., 1985; Earl and Ibbetson, 1986), but the clinician should use a proprietary brand designed for the purpose. Copal varnish and some other varnishes are not effective, although a clear nail varnish may be used. Emolients such as petroleum jelly can be effective, but are not suitable for all clinical situations because they are easily removed by tongue movements. Perhaps the best solution is to use a light-cured bonding agent.

Factors affecting setting characteristics :

There are many chemical and physical factors that affect the setting characteristics of glass-ionomer cements. Although fundamentally an acid-base reaction, the reaction is complicated by the differential release and precipitation of calcium and aluminium ions and by their chelation by fluoride and tartrate ions. While some factors- such as temperature, powder particle size, and powder liquid ratio-merely serve to accelerate or retard the reactions, certain chemical factors have a more profound effect and play an important role in modifying the chemical reaction itself. The two most important are fluoride and tartaric acid.

The role of fluoride :

In their early studies, before the effect of tartaric acid had been discovered, Wilson and Kent had to develop a glass high in fluoride, G-200, in order to obtain any working properties at all. They observed that glasses without fluoride yielded intractable, unworkable pastes. The inference drawn was that the fluoride ion profoundly affected the nature of the cement-forming reaction. Crisp and Wilson (1974a) and Barry and coworkers (1979) demonstrated clearly that working properties were influenced by the amount of fluoride released from the glass. The action of fluoride was attributed to the formation of metal complexes that retarded the binding of cations to anionic sites on the polyelectrolyte chain, thus delaying gelation and prolonging working time. Formation of complexes also releases hydrogen ions, thus increasing the acidity of the paste and delaying pH-dependent gelation.

The effect of tartaric acid:

The favourable effect of fluoride and the knowledge that this effect depended on complex formation prompted Wilson and Crisp to search for other chelating agents (Wilson and Crisp, 1975; Wilson et al., 1976; Crisp and Wilson, 1976). They quickly discovered the unique effectiveness of optically actived tartaric acid (the meso form does not have this effect). This was the key discovery in the development of the glass-ionomer cement as a practical dental material. So important is (+) tartaric acid to the viability of the system, that it must be regarded as a third component.

Tartaric acid is a cement-former in its own right, but its cements are totally unstable toward water (Wilson, 1968; Crisp and Wilson, 1976). But when added in moderate amounts to glass-ionomer cement systems, tartaric acid has several favourable effects. First, it improves manipulation of the cement paste and tends to increase working time. This effect is very noticeable when glasses that do not contain fluoride are used, for the addition of tartaric acid renders workable cement pastes that otherwise would be intractable. Second, tartaric acid sharpens set by accelerating the precipitation process (Crisp and Wilson, 1976). Third, when added in moderate amounts, tartaric acid increases cement strength. More importantly, tartaric acid has vastly widened the range of glasses that can be used for cement formation. Glasses containing less fluoride can be used, laying open the way for developing cements of greater translucency and aesthetic appeal.

The mechanism of action of tartaric acid has not been entirely elucidated, despite the work of Crisp and Wilson (1976) and Prosser and Coworkers (1982a, 1982b). Tartaric acid is a stronger acid than poly (acrylic acid), forming strong complexes with aluminium and so enhancing extraction of aluminium from the glass. Prosser and coworkers (1982b), using carbon-13 nuclear magnetic resonance spectroscopy, showed that the initial reaction is between the glass and tartaric acid. They found initially that tartaric acid alone complexes cations, but then as neutralization proceeds and the pH rises to around 3, poly (acrylic acid) becomes neutralized by metal ions until the cement sets at pH 5.0 to 5.5. In addition, the ionization of poly (acrylic acid) suppressed and the unwinding of the poly (acrylic acid) chain is retarded, thus reducing the viscosity of the paste and delaying gelation. However, once gelation occurs tartaric acid accelerates hardening. Tartaric acid would seem, therefore, to control the initial setting of the cement. Since tartaric acid and calcium react preferentially, the initial set is probably due to the formation of calcium tartrate.

Because glass-ionomer cements that contain tartaric acid are superior in strength to simple glass-ionomer cements, there must be some cooperative interaction between metal ions, tartaric acid, and poly (acrylic acid). Undoubtedly, in the set cement tartrate is incorporated into a molecular structure together with polyacrylate and metal ions. Crisp and Wilson (1976) envisage a cross-linking unit consisting of a pair or metal ions bridged by tartrate that contains two pairs of chelating ligands. It is also possible that fluoride ions are involved in this complex.

Factors affecting the rate of setting:

In previous sections we have shown how certain chemical factors can affect the rate of setting. The effects of some of these-tartaric acid is a case in point can be quite complex. Others are simple physical chemistry effects. Some are controlled in the manufacture and others lie in the hands of the clinician. A list of these factors is given below:

2. Glass composition, especially the alumina/silica ratio and fluoride content. Up to a limiting value, the higher the alumina/silica ratio the faster the set and the shorter the working time.
3. Particle size of the glass powder. The finer the powder the faster the set and the shorter the working time.
4. Addition of tartaric acid. Sharpens the set without shortening the working time.
5. Relative proportions of the constituents in the cement mix, i.e., glass/polyacid / tartaric acid / water. The greater the proportion of glass and the lower the proportion of water the faster the set and the shorter the working time. (Crisp et al, 1976b).
6. Temperature of mixing, The higher the temperature the faster the set and the shorter the working time.

Simple physical chemistry tells us the set will be faster when the powder is finer, the proportion of powder in the mix is greater, the amount of water in the mix is lower, and the temperature of mixing is higher. While a fast set can be an advantage, this is offset by a corresponding loss of working time.

The manufacturer has complete control over glass composition, particle sizes of the glass powder, and the addition of tartaric acid. The temperature of the mix is within the clinician's province and with some materials he can control the powder/ liquid ratio in the mix.

Mclean has, since the early 1970s, employed the technique of chilling the powder and the mixing slab. Mount and Makinson (1978) confirmed the usefulness of this technique and reported an increase in working time without loss of physical properties when slab and powder were cooled. A word of warning: if the liquid is a polyacid solution, chilling it may cause gelation. Also, if the humidity of the environment is high and the temperature of the slab is below the dew point, then moisture will condense on the cement materials and the cement will be weakened. When using this technique it is preferable to use an old-fashioned glass slab because it will have a greater thermal capacity and permit ready observation of moisture condensation when the temperature is below the dew point.

The glass/polyacid/tartaric acid/water ratio is controlled by the manufacturer when the materials are capsulated. For hand-mixed materials control is partly in the hands of the clinician, who can control the powder / liquid ratio. For filling and lining purposes the thickest mix is preferable. Setting, too, is always hastened and strength is improved by increasing the amount of glass powder in the mix. Conversely, setting is delayed and the cement is weakened if the amount of water in the mix is increased.

7. PHYSICAL PROPERTIES OF GLASS-IONOMER CEMENTS:

Setting shrinkage and wear

In resin composite research, a great deal of attention has focused on setting shrinkage because of its importance for sealing composite restorations. Although composites form an acceptable alternative to amalgam for an increasing number of indications, the polymerization shrinkage is still a major problem. As a result of contraction during the setting stage, loss of adhesion to the cavity walls may occur where the tensile shrinkage stresses on the adhesive bonds reach levels that surpass the bond strength.

Setting shrinkage of glass ionomers is equally important, because these materials may be used as an alternative to composites.

While a property such as setting shrinkage is mainly concerned with the clinical success of a restoration in terms of retention and sealing, the longevity of the surface contour is determined by the restorative material's resistance to wear.

Setting Shrinkage of Glass-ionomers

To facilitate the discussion, the setting processes for the different types of glass-ionomers are summarized first.

Setting of conventional glass-ionomers

The setting of conventional glass-ionomer cements starts when the liquid and powder are brought into contact with each other. This produces an acid-base- reaction in which the acid is a poly-alkenoic (eg, polyacrylic or polymaleic) acid, and the base is a finely powdered glass consisting of fluoroaluminosilicates. The polyacid is either part of the liquid as an aqueous solution or incorporated into the powder in a freeze-dried state. In the latter case, the liquid is simply water in which the freeze-dried polyacid dissolves on mixing.

The hydrogen ions of the acid penetrate the glass particles and release calcium, strontium, and aluminum ions, which combine with the polyalkenoic chains of the acid to form an initial rubbery hydrogel structure. In the following phase of the setting reaction, the metal ions form cross-links between the polyalkenoic chains, creating a highly rigid material. This portion of the reaction may continue over a period of weeks or even months. During all stages of the reaction and also in the set state, all these materials are sensitive to dehydration.

Setting of resin-modified glass-ionomers

The slow rate of setting and the sensitivity to dehydration of conventional glass-ionomer cements are unfavorable properties in comparison with resin composites. In an attempt to overcome these disadvantages, hybrid material were developed that combine resin composite and conventional glass-ionomer technologies. These resin-modified glass-ionomers are light curable and less sensitive to dehydration, while retaining most of the advantages of conventional glass-ionomers. Some of these material are now widely used in such products as Fuji II LC, Photac-Fil, and Vitremer. They are derived from conventional glass-ionomer cements, in which part of the water content is replaced by the water-soluble and photopolymerizable 2-hydroxyethylmethacrylate (HEMA) monomer.

The setting of resin-modified glass-ionomers involves the polymerization of the HEMA monomer by light activation and the classic acid-base reaction between a polyacid and the basic glass particles. However, in many cases the monomer will polymerize even without light because the manufacturer has added a catalyst to the composition.

The rubbery hydrogel phase seen with conventional glass ionomers is not expressed after light curing. This is because the polymerization reaction of the monomer rapidly lends the material considerable strength. The acid-base reaction proceeds within the polymer network that has been formed, and the two reactions ultimately result in the formation of two interpenetrating matrices.

MAS-NMR spectroscopy studies in the setting reaction of glass ionomer cements:

Hill and co-authors have developed a series of glass compositions (4.5SiO2–3Al2O3 1.5P2O5–(5 z)CaO–zCaF2), that can crystallise to both apatite and mullite with appropriate heat treatment and the resultedglass ceramics exhibit high fracture toughness. The presence of fluorine is essential for the formation of the crystalline apatite phase. On the other hand, lack of fluorine results in a tricalcium phosphate crystalline phase. The crystallization process of the above series of glasses has been extensively investigated leading to the conclusion that both fluoride content and CaO/P2O5 ratio play an important role in the crystallisation of the apatite phase.Recently, magic angle spinning nuclear magnetic resonance (MAS-NMR) spectroscopy has been successfully applied for the structural analysis of both crystalline and amorphous glass solids of alumino-silicate and silicate compounds. 19F MAS-NMR spectroscopy10 has shown that in high fluorine containing glasses, the fluorine present in the F–Ca(n) environment within the glass is used preferentially in forming the fluorapatite crystalline phase already at the first crystallization peak temperature whereas the Al–F–Ca(n) species present in the glass start disappearing only at the second crystallisation peak temperature. The composition of these glasses is very close to the glass compositions used for the commercial glass ionomer cements and their use in forming glass ionomer cements has also been investigated. It has been reported, that the properties of glass ionomer cements are influenced by the glass composition, for example the Al/Si and Ca/P ratios, the fluorite and fluorine content. In addition, the substitution of oxygen for fluorine results in significantly decreasing the setting time even at low fluorine concentrations. On the other hand, the compressive strength of cements increases when the concentration of fluorine is low and it is not significantly affected when the concentration of fluorine in the glass is high.[37]

Although the setting reaction in glass ionomer cements has been extensively studied, the setting process of the cements has not been yet fully understood.In a MAS-MNR study the Al spectra showed clearly the formation of six-fold coordinate Al(VI), that may crosslink the carboxyl groups in the poly-acid molecules. A shift towards to more positive values of the carboxyl peak in the C CP/MAS-NMR spectra showed clearly the proton dissociation of the carboxyl groups. A shift towards more negative values was observed in the Si MAS-NMR spectra, suggesting formation of hydrated silica gel and consequently formation of additional Si–O–Si bonds. MAS-NMR spectra also reflected changes in the coordination state around a PO4 tetrahedron. Increasing the fluorine content of the glasses resulted generally in increased reactivity during setting, due to promoting cross-linking and repolymerisation of the silicate phase, followed by clear changes in the MAS-NMR spectra. The cross-linking process during the setting reaction of glass ionomer cements can be followed by MAS-NMR spectroscopy observing the conversion of Al(IV) to Al(VI). The acid base setting reaction is completed in 1 day and no further significant changes in the MAS-NMR spectra can be observed. Further study is required in order to understand the role of phosphorus.[37]

Setting shrinkage

Using measuring devices, which make it possible to determine the dimensional changes, which take place during the setting of restorative materials (such as the mercury dilatometer), it has been demonstrated that both types of glass-ionomer cements undergo considerable setting shrinkage. In the case of resin-modified glass-ionomers, shrinkage occurs for both the polymerization reaction of the monomers and the acid-base reaction, depending on the moment of light activation. For example, when light activation is started within 2 minutes after mixing, shrinkage occurs only for the polymerization reaction. No shrinkage of the acid-base reaction can take place, because it is completely blocked by the polymer network. However, when light activation is omitted or delayed for a time, the shrinkage of the acid-base reaction can be expressed during this period. If the manufacturer has included a catalyst in the composition for the polymerization of the monomer, there is a contributory shrinkage effect as a result of the chemically initiated polymerization reaction. The extent of the ultimate shrinkage when light activation is delayed or omitted is different for each resin modified material. It is important to note that resin-modified glass-ionomers also cure in the absence of light activation. This is known as the dark curing of resin-modified glass-ionomers. The process generally proceeds slowly, but if a situation occurs that prevents the light from the light source reaching deep parts of a restoration, curing ultimately takes place[36]

. **Setting shrinkage of different types of glass ionmers**

Material	Type	Manufacturer	Setting Shrinkage (vol%)
Ketac-Fil Aplicap	Conventional	Espe	3.4
Ketac-Molar	Conventional	Espe	4.4
Fuji II Capsule	Conventional	GC	3.6
Fuji IX Capsule	Conventional	GC	3.6
Chem-Fil Superior	Conventional	DeTrey/Dentsply	4.1
Shofu Hi-Dense	Metal-modified	Shofu	2.6
Miracle Mix	Metal-modified	GC	3.5
Ketac-Silver	Metal-modified	Espe	3.1
Photac-Fil Aplicap	Resin-modified	Espe	3.8
Fuji II LC Capsule	Resin-modified	GC	4.8
Vitremer	Resin-modified	3M	4.3

Shrinkage stress in bonded restorations

In a restoration that is adhesively bonds to the cavity walls, the material exerts tensile stress on the walls during setting. The ultimate extent of the shrinkage stress in a cavity determines whether bonding to the cavity wall is retained.

One of the most important factor & influencing the degree of stress is the shape of the cavity. The larger the surface of the cavity walls to which the restoration bonds, the greater the stress. Conversely a fairly large unbonded surface keeps the shrinkage stress low, because a relatively large amount of material from the free surface is able to flow to the stress area. Thus, the final shrinkage stress depends, on the geometry of the cavity preparation.

With the aid of a simulation model, the details of which are not presented here, it is possible to study the development of shrinkage stress during setting for any cavity geometry[36].experiments with this model show that the shrinkage stress developed by glass-ionomer cements is considerably lower than that of resin composites, despite the fact that glass-ionomer cements display a much higher setting shrinkage than do composites (2.0 to 3.0 vol%). In the case of simulated shallow Class V restoration, stresses in composites can reach values of 15-18 MPa, whereas those for conventional and resin-modified glass- ionomers do not exceed 2 to 3 MPa. Thus, there is a strong possibility that a Class V composite restoration will detach from the cavity wall during setting, because the shrinkage stresses may exceed the bond strength.

The low shrinkage stress of conventional glass-ionomer cements is due largely to the rubbery stage these cements pass through during the setting process. Besides flow, elastic yielding also relieves the shrinkage stress. When both factors are favorable, there is a strong possibility that the bonding to the cavity walls, which is approximately 6 MPa for enamel and 3 MPa for dentin, will be retained during setting. However, when the material is subject to dehydration, adhesive or cohesive failure may occur.

The shrinkage stresses recorded for resin-modified glass-ionomers are some- what higher than those of the conventional materials. This is due to the fact that the shrinkage is totally dominated by the light-initiated polymerization reaction. No rubbery phase can be distinguished, as in the case of the acid-base reaction. Therefore, the shrinkage stresses do not experience elastic relaxation. In most materials the degree of shrinkage stress following light activation is approximately 3 MPa. It is not surprising that the stresses are again lower than the 18 MPa recorded for light-curing composites, because the amount of monomer in resin-modified glass-ionomers is only 3% as opposed to 30% to 50% in composites. As yet, little is known about the effect of shrinkage stress on the bonding of the restoration to the cavity wall, but leakage tests have shown that resin-modified materials are comparable to conventional cements in this respect.

Water sorption and relaxation of setting stresses:

It is generally assumed that shrinkage stress can be wholly or partially counteracted by hygroscopic expansion as a result of water sorption. The solid curves in Fig2-1 show what happens when contact with water occurs after 15 minutes. The stress decreases almost immediately, but then increases again. The decrease shows that glass-ionomer cements are capable of absorbing water and that this occurs quite rapidly. The stress then increases, due to the advanced stage of the reaction, so the development of shrinkage stresses again predominates. From this moment, however, hygroscopic expansion actively opposes shrinkage stress. This is particularly evident in the upper curves in. There it continues to rise because the materials have not been brought into contact with water. It may be concluded from this experiment that as soon as wet finishing in the mouth begins, the development of shrinkage stress is slowed by water sorption.

An unexpected result is that total relaxation is not attained within a period of 14 hours. A downward trend is visible, and it is possible that this process lasts for several days.

The interaction between resin-based cement and water involves two opposing phenomena. On the one hand, water will leach out unreacted monomers and other species), contributing to shrinkage, loss in weight, and reduction of mechanical properties1). On the other hand, water sorption leads to a swelling of the material and an increase in weight. The use of resin-based cements under restorations has been implicated in the subsequent fracture of the latter. In an *in vitro* study, it was shown that restorations which were cemented to extracted teeth and which were exposed to deionized water eventually fractured[38].

In the case of resin-modified glass-ionomers, hygroscopic expansion also occurs following exposure to water. Total relaxation is attained within 5 hours and from that point the reverse process takes is place, building up expansion forces. Nevertheless:, any marginal crevice that may appear as a result of shrinkage stress does not achieve a perfect attachment, because the planes of fracture will never fit together as perfectly as before.

After 14 hours the expansion has still not come to an end and may continue for a long time. Obviously, the ultimate compressive stress must not be too high, because this can lead to cracks in the tooth material.

In contrast to conventional cements the omission of water contact does not necessarily lead to cohesive or adhesive failure in resin-modified materials, but shrinkage stresses continue to increase. In the clinical situation, contact with water almost always takes place directly after setting by light activation, which occurs within 5 minutes study examined the solubility, sorption, and dimensional change of eight luting cements in two different solutions:

50% ethanol:water and distilled water

The values of water sorption (Wso) and solubility (Wsl) were calculated using the following equations(ISO 4049:2000):

$$Wso = \frac{m1 - m2}{V}$$

$$Wsl = \frac{m0 - m2}{V}$$

m0 is the specimen mass before immersion (mg), m1 is the specimen mass after immersion, m2 is the specimen mass after desiccation (mg), and V is the specimen volume before immersion (mm3).

For each group, the means and standard deviations for solubility, sorption (μg/mm3), and change in percentage volume were calculated. This study demonstrated that in both water and ethanol:water solution, resin-modified glass ionomer cements exhibited higher sorption and solubility as compared to resin-based luting cements. Among the resin-based luting cements, higher water sorption was exhibited by the cement with a lower filler content.

The resin-modified glass ionomer cements exhibited lower sorption in ethanol than in water. On the contrary, resin-based cements exhibited higher sorption in ethanol than in water.

Sorption and solubility values were found to depend on the type and content of filler, filler concentration, mean particle size, the coupling agents, the nature of the filler particles, and the type of solvent[38].

Wear of Glass-Ionomers

Although the loss of substance displayed by restorations in the occlusal area is caused by a number of wear mechanisms occlusal wear is thought to be primarily three-body in nature. This type of wear results from the abrasive activity of solid particles in a food bolus when it is pressed onto and sheared across the occlusal surfaces of opposing teeth during mastication. Lutz et al have described this as wear in the occlusal contact-free areas (CFA). The wear resulting from direct contact is defined as wear in the occlusal contact area (OCA), which involves such mechanisms as two body abrasive wear, adhesive wear, a surface fatigue. Another type of wear is corrosive in nature, where chemical factors soften or degrade the surface of the restoration.

Although it is only in the mouth that the wear mechanisms described come into play simultaneously and thus interacts with each other, some of the wear component can be imitated simultaneously or separtely using the ACTA wear machine. Research has demonstrated that the machine not only makes possible a good simulation of clinical CFA, but also provides an impression of the wear caused by surface fatigue in the OCA. The role of chemical components, such as acids, also can be studied.

Characteristics of wear

Due to their limited mechanical strength brittleness, and high degree of wear, applications of glass-ionomer cement have thus far been limited to erosion and abrasion lesions, or Class III and Class V cavities. Metal-modified cements, including cermets, have been employed occlusally in primary molars with varying degrees of success and in permanen teeth where chewing stresses are low.

The limited wear resistance of glass-ionomer cements on chewing surfaces thought to be due to insufficient strength directly after placement. It is only after the cements have had time to build up greater degree of strength that wear resistance reaches an acceptable level. This increase in mechanical properties may take weeks or even months.

Another factor that may influence wear resistance is the sensitivity to acids. This is liable to be a problem in those areas where mechanical forces and acids are active at the same time, such as on occlusal surfaces during mastication of acidic food substances.

Despite the general view that glass-ionomers are not yet suitable for occlusal applications, the temptation to use them has often been too great to resist. With the advent of resin-modified glass-ionomer cements, which appear to set fully after light activation, an occlusal filling is often considered an attractive option.

The rest of this section examines the wear performance of conventional, metal- modified, and resin-modified glass-ionomers in contact-free and occlusal contact areas during the early stages after placement and in the long-term, as well as the susceptibility of these materials to acids as studied using the ACTA wear machine.

Early and long-term wear of glass-ionomer cements

Unlike composite resins, in which the polymerization reaction ceases within a week after initiation, the setting process for all types of glass-ionomers continues over a period of several months. This is reflected in the high early wear rates determined directly after preparation of the samples, and the declining wear over time. Even between 4 months and 1 year there is evidence of a reduction in wear. The continuing improvement in mechanical properties is probably the result of the slow displacement of calcium ions by aluminum ions, which further enhances the cohesion of the matrix.

The wear of resin-modified glass-ionomers appears to be significantly higher than that of the conventional materials, probably due to differences in matrix formation. The matrix of a conventional glass-ionomer consists of an ionically cross-linked polyalkenoate network resulting from an acid-base reaction. The set cements of resin- modified Photac-Fil and Fuji II LC have similar cross-linked polyalkenoate networks, but these are entangled with HEMA polymer chains. In the case of Vitremer, the polyalkenoate network and polymer chains are connected through pendant methacrylate groups on the polyalkenoate chains. The greater wear displayed by resin-modified materials may indicate that the coherence of filler particles embedded in the interpenetrating matrices of polyalkenoate and polymer is inferior to that of the particles in the conventional matrix. This may be due to the partial replacement of the rigid polyalkenoate network by the flexible polymer chains. The increased deformation of the surface caused by the load of mastication, as simulated in the wear machine, can lead to the formation of subsurface microcracks in the ionic cross- linked polyalkenoate matrix with a subsequent loss of coherence.

In fact, this type of wear is related to subsurface fatigue, which takes on dramatic proportions under the conditions prevailing at occlusal contact areas. While Photac-Fil and Fuji II LC show an approximate increase in wear of 200% from CFA to OCA, the increase is limited to 50% in the case of Vitremer. The superior performance of Vitremer indicates that the chemical integration of its two matrices leads to a higher stability than a coherence based on entanglement. Also, the conventional glass-ionomers, with the exception of Ketac- Silver, are more sensitive at occlusal contacts as simulated in the wear machine, but the wear on these materials , increases by only about 30%.

It is noteworthy that the metal-modified Ketac-Silver cermet, which is indicated for use on occlusal surfaces in primary molars, does not perform any better with respect to long-term CFA wear than Keta Fil. Thus, the superior clinical performance of Ketac-Silver must be due to its more favorable early CFA wear and its higher resistance to OCA wear. In this respect, the high viscous Ketac-Molar and Fuji IX also show better performance than their predecessors, Ketac-Fil and Fuji II.

Wear under acidic conditions.

Acids directly attack the surface of glass-ionomers, causing the dissolution of the cement. The extent to which this occurs depends on the degree of acidity. When acids and wear mechanisms operate simultaneously, as on occlusal areas during mastication of acidic food substances or directly after consumption of acidic drinks, their influence is noticeable at a pH as low as 5. The material's degree of sensitivity to acid is considered important, because it may be one of the factors, contributing to clinical durability. A test that is commonly used to determine the acid sensitivity of cements is the lactic acid jet test. Cement surfaces are exposed to a powerful jet comprising solution of lactic acid in water which has pH of 4. The classification of conventional and metal-modified glass-ionomer cements with respect to acid sensitivity as determined by this test corresponds to the decrease in wear under acid conditions in the ACTA wear machine: Fuji II= Shofu Hi-Dense < Chem-Fil Superior < ketac-Fil < Ketac-Silver.

Tests for the stability of resin-modified glass-ionomers under acidic condition resulted in interesting finding which have not yet been explained. It would appear that the presence of the resin is sufficient to provide a certain degree of protection against acid. It is possible that in the early stages after setting this category of materials is sensitive to pH values of 5 or lower, as has been demonstrated for comparable cements such as Vitrebond and XR-ionomer at pH 4 using the lactic acid jet test.

It is clear from the marked degree of early CFA wear (> 100µm) compared to that of resin composites (30 to 60 µm) that resin-modified materials are not yet suitable for occlusal restorations. However, some glass-ionomers, such as conventional Ketac-Fil and metal-modified Shofu Hi-Dense, may be able to compete with composites as their long-term wear falls in the 20 to 50µm range. Moreover, because of the high intra-oral temperature, setting in the mouth is expected to proceed more rapidly, so that under clinical conditions a higher wear resistance will be attained sooner.

Table 2-3 Contact-free area wear of glass-ionomers directly after preparation and finishing and in the long term as determined with the ACTA wear machine

Material	Type	Manufacturer	Wear (µm)		
			1 day	4 months	1 year
Ketac-Fil Aplicap	Conventional	Espe	116	35	30
Ketac-Molar	Conventional	Espe	88	42	36
Fuji II Capsule	Conventional	GC	167	65	57
Fuji IX Capsule	Conventional	GC	119	57	51
Chem-Fil Superior	Conventional	DeTrey/Dentsply	128	58	53
Shofu Hi-Dense	Metal-modified	Shofu	116	32	27
Miracle Mix	Metal-modified	GC	154	65	48
Ketac-Silver	Metal-modified	Espe	95	64	52
Photac-Fil Aplicap	Resin-modified	Espe	522	172	152
Fuji II LC Capsule	Resin-modified	GC	308	155	138
Vitremer	Resin-modified	3M	211	90	82

Fatigue and elasticity

The clinical application of restorative materials has always been preceded by extensive laboratory research into their physical and mechanical properties. This is true for glass-ionomer cements.

Elements of Fatigue Behavior

Stiffness and wear resistance

Stiffness has long been one of the primary focuses in dental material research. The advantage of studying this property is that a quick, straightforward methodology can easily be used to study the influence of a variety of test and by environmental variables. Whereas studies of stiffness initially were used mainly in a purely quantitative way, this property has gradually evolved into a verification instrument for qualitative information such as elasticity gradients in hybrid layers.

Such an approach can only be used if one accepts that it is impossible to use a single parameter, or even a combination of parameters, quantitatively to predict more complex processes, such as wear. As a consequence, research has been initiated to study complex processes as quasi-solitary phenomena, mainly by trying to imitate and simulate the clinical environment, which restorative materials need to function properly. Gradually, the influence of diverse individual factors such as chewing force and the composition of the saliva can be sorted out, while the simulator is normalized using the results of clinical studies. In this way researchers can gain insight into the different types of wear occurring under simulated clinical conditions. In dentistry, the loss of material due to non-antagonistic contacts has been defined as occlusal contact-free area (CFA) wear. Occlusal contact area (OCA) wear has been designated as material loss caused by direct interaction of an antagonist with the restorative material. For one major group of restoratives, resin composites, CFA wear is no longer considered a problem. Also, most of these materials have highly improved OCA wear, with some showing wear resistance equal to that of amalgam. However, in spite of excellent wear resistance, some restorations fail all of a sudden. therefore, something else must come into play; fatigue.

Fatigue

As with wear, *fatigue* is only a nonspecific descriptive term that stands for several different expressions damage accumulation inside a material caused by static fatigue conditions, dynamic and/or cyclic fatigue. They all have one basic feature in common: crack growth.

Studying wear phenomena occurring under OCA conditions emphasizes the presence of cracks in both the wear facet itself and its immediate vicinity. This lends credence to the hypothesis that there is something like fatigue wear, which causes a delamination of wear particles following subsurface crack growth in situations where there is cyclic sliding of a plunger on a test surface (eg, an antagonistic cusp on the surface of a filling). Such subsurface cracks have been identified both in vitro and in vivo.

Given that wear and fatigue seem to be related, at least by the basic underlying damage mechanism, it becomes of primary importance to study a cement's crack sensitivity or its reciprocal, crack resistance, together with the influences on the clinical environment on this property. It must be realized that the corrosive action of oral fluids, certainly in cements and even in polymers, may contribute significantly to the crack growth sensitivity of a material.

However, even for traditional engineering materials such as metals, for which fatigue has been a recognized problem for decades, the fundamental causes of failure are not yet completely understood therefore, one can readily accept that materials such as dental resin composites and cements, the era of fatigue studies just started and that fatigue data are only sparsely available. Although current knowledge on the fatigue behavior of trials, such as fiber-reinforced composites, is growing rapidly, it is highly unlike that the same effort will be directed toward the relatively small market of dental restoratives. [4]

Furthermore, despite the volume of work undertaken to discover the fatigue properties of plastics, very little effort is being made to design standardized methods. As a consequence, standard developed in fatigue testing of metals have been adapted for use with plastics, although extreme care must be exercise because metals behave differently than do viscoelastic plastics. Furthermore, the fatigue properties of plastics are often influenced to a large extent by the environment in which they are used and/or tested. This certainly holds true for dental restorative materials.

The present situation points to necessity of establishing standardized testing and gathering fatigue data for dental restorative materials, thereby allowing a better understanding of the major failure processes of wear and fatigue. However, strength also is a factor in failures of restorations and should integrated with wear and fatigue as object of study.

Strength

Two types of loading conditions cause a material to lose strength over time. The first is static loading in the presence of chemical agent, and the second is cyclic loading. It is obvious that both conditions occur simultaneously in the mouth, and that one can speak about cyclic loading in chemically active environment.

Under cyclic stress (eg, in extension), a material may fail at stresses well below its known ultimate stress limit. Often tens of thousands of cycles will elapse without incident, followed by a rapid and sudden catastrophic failure, as has been described in the literature for microfilled composites. In general, the higher the stress, the shorter the life of the restoation. Furthermore, composition and chemical structure, as well as environmental conditions, exert profound influence on mechanically induced crack propagation.

Fatigue failure involves two mechanisms: weakening due to energy-dissipating modes of relaxation, and mechanical initiation and propagation of a crack. The latter mechanism is especially dominant at low frequencies, as in the mouth where generally a chewing frequency of 1 to 2Hz is present. A simple fatigue scenario would then be a progressive loss of strength due to the gradual spread of one or more cracks. Fatigue is the growth of these cracks under cyclic loading conditions. Thus, it is necessary to find out why cracks develop and grow.

In most if not all materials, the onset of crack growth initiates from a preexisting flaw or defect. In dental ceramics, intrinsic effects may arise from microstructural features, whereas extrinsic defects may be introduced by grinding during occlusal adjustment. One must also take into consideration that crack growth may be complicated by crack healing or blunting of the crack tip during prolonged nonstressed periods.

In composite materials, frictional sliding or debonding between the reinforced phase and the matrix also may occur. In the latter case, the effect of an aqueous environment on subcritical crack growth and mechanical degradation will be profound: silicate glasses are among the most (corrosive) fatigue-susceptible of all ceramics. Furthermore, although voids can be helpful in the reduction of curing stresses, they are also structural imperfections that encourage crack growth.

Evaluation of Glass-Ionomers for Fatigue

Glass-ionomer cements are considered particle-reinforced materials. The generally low strength of conventional glass-ionomers can be explained by a mismatch in the mechanical properties of the glass-ionomer matrix and the glass particles, causing large stresses to accumulate at the interface. Numerous voids can be detected in these materials. The voids vary substantially in size and diameter, depending on the processing method followed. In metal-reinforced glass-ionomers, the well-bonded, high- strength discrete metal particles may act as pinning sites of the crack front, thus retarding crack growth, perhaps altogether. It is not yet known what the effect of the added resinous components in resin-modified glass-ionomers may be in terms of fatigue behavior. There also is little to nothing known about the behavior of polyacid-modified composites, also called compomers. The rest of this section discusses to test for fatigue behavior. The focus is on one particular study involving composites and glass-ionomer cements.

Testing techniques

One way of studying crack growth creating test samples that contain an artificially induced crack of known length. This can be achieved rather through polymerization of a material against a sharp raiser knife or by indentation. The disadvantage of this technique is that an artificial crack cannot truly mimic naturally occurring defects caused by processing, occlusal adjustment, or occlusal forces. Furthermore, although the artificial crack tends grow in a constant direction, real fatigue can deviate significantly from their normal and expected growth plane due to interactions of the crack tip with microstructural inhomogeneities, environmental elements, and other factors. Fracture toughness tests, which have been carried out on many composite resin materials, use this methodology.

Indents can be produced with hardness indenters, and this type of experiment has been used to study composites and porcelains. Results with polymeric materials all indicate that the presence of an aqueous environment yields to plasticizing of the matrix phase, thereby lowering most mechanical properties. When indenters that mimic the tips of natural tooth cusps are used, it is found that the matrix phase can undergo considerable plastic deformation without failure. It also has been shown that cracks can be formed at loads of about 50N, which are easily achieved during mastication.[40]

Unfortunately, all these tests lack effect of cyclic loading. It might be expected that cyclic loading is harmful to a material than steady loading because the average deflection over the cyclic period is less than the steady deflection. However, it is the cyclically loaded material that breaks and the statically loaded one that survives. So, inspite of the important knowledge that material be gathered from static and dynamic fatigue tests, they must be combined with data obtained from cyclic fatigue test's. a common way to establish the fatigue behavior of materials is by studying the number of cycles survived at different stresses, the Wohler curve.

Fracture is the final fatigue criterion that needs to be included in testing. However, this is not possible for the study of cyclic fatigue in particulate-reinforced materials, which have widely varying compositions resulting generally in anisotropic behavior. Furthermore, the establishment of a fatigue criterion becomes complicated due to the several modes of damage accumulation. Therefore, most fatigue criteria for such materials are dictated by the application area of the structure or the specific properties of material itself; for example, the percentage of stiffness loss at an establishd point of fiber and matrix composition can be used. Models for the mathematical approach of measuring fatigue in composites are not readily available; often, the analytical approach is based on linear fracture mechanics, which may or may not apply to glass-ionomer cements. Because many dental materials are heterogeneous in structure and are likely to contain faults or imperfections such as porosity in varying amounts and sizes, the time taken for crack propagation and fracture or material loss by wear is expected to vary considerably. However, at this time, more appropriate equations have not been reported.[4]

One could conclude that each group of materials seems to fail by mechanisms specific to that group, and generalizations are hard to make. Rather than looking for the absolute answer in terms of fatigue behavior, a more interesting approach may be to study different dental restoratives under identical testing conditions, which ideally should resemble the clinical service environment. Experimentally, there are several valid approaches.

First, a series of tests can be performed at various levels of stress, and the number of cycles survived can be observed. This Wohler-type of experiment requires many samples and a lot of time. Another approach is to compare the relative levels of stress at which different materials can survive for a pre-set number of stress cycles. This approach is often referred to as a *staircase method.* Tests are conducted sequentially with the maximum applied stress in each test being increased or decreased by a fixed increment, according to whether the previous test resulted in failure or non- failure.

A comparable method is the *boundary method,* which has some advantages over the staircase method. It is less time consuming if more than one testing machine is available. Once suitable load levels have been selected, it also allows for simultaneous testing, unlike the staircase method, in which the outcome of anyone test must be known before the next can be started.

Materials and methods

Based on the preceding review, a fatigue test was developed[43] using a staircase methodology, with the pre-set number of cycles at 10,000 Samples were tested in a stress-controlled mode at a test frequency of 2 Hz. Dynamic creep was compensated for by clamping of the samples. Prior to fatigue testing, the clamped fracture strength was determined (n = 6), and the amount of increase or decrease of fatigue stress following non-failure or failure, respectively, was arbitrarily set at 4% of this strength. Tests were performed at 35°C.

After preparation, samples were stored for 1 month, either dry (n = 12) or in distilled water (n = 12), at 35°C. In an additional test, freshly prepared samples (n = 12) for selected products were subjected to the fatigue regimen under wet testing conditions, and the fatigue limit was immediately determined. The samples that did not fail were tested again after 1 month of wet storage.

Representative composites, conventional glass-ionomers, resin-modified glass ionomers, and polyacid-modified composites were evaluated.

Results

In general, for all composite materials tested, the flexural fatigue limit (FFL) after water sorption was significantly lower. This was also the case for the glass-ionomer HiFi Master Palette. It was not true for Shofu FX, the resin-modified glass-ionomers, or the polyacid-modified composite.

The results for the immediate fatigue reveal that all materials tested showed significant decrease in FFL at 5 minute compared to the dry FFL. When examining the wet FFL, all materials but the composites had a significantly decreased FFL, with the resin-modified glass-ionomers scoring only about 50%. One month later, however, only Z100 had a significantly lower FFL than the wet samples.

The investigation into fractured surfaces revealed several common fracture characteristics. Regardless of the type of material tested, most often the fracture was initiated at an inclusion or imperfection: a void, a filler particle, and so on. In the microfilled materials, markings of the cyclic nature of crack growth could be identified clearly at both the filler particles and the matrix phase. The crack retardation effect of optimal particle size distribution on crack growth also could be seen.

Discussion :

Water plays a major role in filler-matrix bond failures in resin-based matrices. It leaches out filler elements; it induces filler failures and filler-matrix debonding, thereby reducing the strength of the matrix material because debonded fillers may act as stress concentrators and significantly multiply the number of potential crack growth sites; and it has a plasticizing effect on the matrix. Therefore, it is extremely important that fatigue tests are run in a humid environment, in which composites are immersed in water for at least 30 days. The present results show that water decreased the flexural fatigue limits of the tested composite materials.

The hydrophilic 2-hydroxyethylmethacrylate (HEMA) is used in most resin- modified glass-ionomers, at a concentration of about 5% in the final set material. Neither version of Fuji II LC or of Vitremer deteriorated after water sorption, thus supporting the hypothesis that "self-healing" or "repair" could be possible in glass-ionomer cements.26 However, this healing may be a retardation in crack growth or a crack growth toughening mechanism, possibly due to the plasticizing effect of the resinous component.

The results for conventional glass-ionomers add to the controversy about the influence of time and water on their properties. A decline following exposure to an aqueous environment is attributed to the plasticizing and erosive effect of water on the cement, as reviewed by Gladys. A healing mechanism is apparently not present in HiFi Master Palette because its fatigue resistance decreased 13.5% after water uptake. It is suggested that extrinsic water inhibits the matrix-forming process of a conventional glass-ionomer, leading to a strength reduction.[44]

In Dyract, the acidic polymerizable monomer (tetracarboxylbutane) has two methacrylate groups, as well as two carboxyl groups, and accounts for about 28% of the composition (technical information from DeTrey/Dentsply). This monomer not only can cross-link when initiated through radical polymerization, but also undergoes an acid-base reaction with the reactive glass particles if water is absorbed from the tooth and the oral environment. This is reflected in the results where Dyract performs better than the other composites tested. In the dry storage samples, the postpolymerization predominated over the acid-base reaction, and was even reinforced by storage in the oven at 35°C. Once placed in a wet environment, the active carboxylic groups undergo the acid-base reaction. This delayed reaction may compensate for the plasticizing effect of water on the resin component.

The fatigue results of the freshly prepared samples show that the composites tested already have a flexural fatigue limit after about 5 minutes, comparable to that after 1 month of undisturbed postcuring in wet storage conditions. After 1 month, however, there are significant differences among the products tested.

The microfilled composite has not suffered from the stress applied during the initial formation of the cross-linked polymer network. The hybrid composite however, clearly shows evidence of loss in fatigue resistance, probably due to damage encountered during the first fatigue test at 5 minutes, which then created opportunities for water to further attack the weakened material. Because the hybrid composite is highly filled, at some spots the matrix remaining between the filler particles became too vulnerable with regard to fatigue stresses.

The resin-modified glass-ionomers showed a remarkable increase in fatigue resistance 1 month after the immediate fatigue test, resulting in a fatigue resistance that was no different from that obtained under unstressed storage conditions. Thus, the acid-base reaction continued following water uptake.[44]

The polyacid-modified material also did not suffer from the imposed fatigue regimen immediately after curing. It is not clear whether this can be attributed strictly to postcuring of the resinous matrix or the continued acid-base reaction, or to a combination of both factors.

Most fatigue tests apply a given load at a given stress rate without taking into account the stress state of the tested surface. Only a few studies have determined the actual fatigue stress. Indeed, a load of 100 N may result in a stress of 10 MPa with a surface contact surface of 10 mm^2 versus 1 MPa for a contact surface of 100 mm^2. Thus, it is important to know the stress limits to which fillings will be subjected during clinical service.

The maximum biting force varies between 108 and 608 N for natural teeth, with the greatest forces exhibited by the molars. The forces used during mastication show peak values of 32 to 374 N, with an average of about 20 N. These values may differ substantially during the chewing cycle and the progressive reduction in the size of food particles. Generally, the load remains smaller during 95% of the chewing cycle. When the load rises, the functional maximal values are about 71 N. The force exerted on the teeth during swallowing is, on average, twice the force exerted during mastication. These values are, of course, force values and should be considered as forces exerted on a surface. To be able to calculate the stress at the occlusal contact area, one must consider the surface area of an antagonistic cusp, which can be estimated at about 1 mm2. The average stress state of a restorative under antagonistic load can be estimated at between 10 to 20 MPa, with short peaks of about 70 MPa during chewing. Consequently, the stress increases from 40 MPa up to 160 MPa during swallowing.

It is interesting to note that some work using finite element analysis with an applied load of 100 N at 90 degrees to the internal inclined plane of the buccal cusp, reports tensile stresses in the filling of 12.4, 22.5, and 42.5 MPa, ranging up to 82.5 MPa.

After wet storage, conventional glass- ionomers score below the arbitrary 40 MPa criterion. Even more important is that resin-modified materials seem to be very vulnerable at the early stages of placement, with a fatigue resistance of about 25 MPa. Thus, it must be remembered that one of the primary characteristics of fatigue is that a material will fail at stresses below its static strength.

Conclusion :

The fatigue resistance of resin-modified glass ionomers after water sorption is between that of microfilled composites and polyacid-modified composites. Resin- modified composites, however, seem to be vulnerable at the early stages after curing, although this is not reflected in the fatigue behavior at later stages. Fatigue resistance is still a matter of concern and stress-bearing restorations should, therefore, be avoided. Hybrid composites also can be vulnerable during early fatigue stresses, probably due to their high filler content.

Elasticity

As stated at the beginning, it is important to have a good understanding of the underlying principles that rule the properties of restorative materials. One of these principles is that mechanical and physical properties originate from a material's internal structure, which involves atoms and the way these atoms are associated with their neighbors. This internal structure may be altered when the material is deformed.

Under clinical circumstances, fillings are put under stress in a chemically active environment with superimposed thermal fluctuations. As a consequence, properties change. Some changes can be spotted easily, such as wear and failure to which have already been discussed. These changes are symptoms, expressing that the internal structure has been modified due to applied stimuli. It is of interest, therefore, to study a property that is capable of reflecting the internal structure of materials and the changes structure undergoes: elasticity.

The modulus of elasticity

One of the few principal properties capable of providing a basis for understanding the relationship between structure and properties is Young's modulus, or the modulus of elasticity. This property can be derived from the stress-strain characteristics of a given material.

Stress is the measure of force per unit area. Strain is the dimensional response to this stress. Plastic strain occurs when the stress exceeds a critical value that initiates a permanent displacement of atoms from their neighbors and, therefore, is irreversible. Elastic strain is reversible; when the stress is removed, the strain disappears. Elastic strain is commonly a clear function of stress. The modulus relating unidirectional elastic strain and stress is the modulus of elasticity (E).

The modulus of elasticity also reflects the strain capacity of a given material, acting more or less as the reciprocal of the modulus itself. The higher the modulus of elasticity, the lower the strain capacity within certain limits.

Clinical Considerations

Many studies have shown that it is difficult to obtain a proper and lasting seal of the cervical border for a cavity filled with resin composite, especially when this border is situated in dentin. This is mainly due to the polymerization shrinkage of the composite toward the enamel, where a string bond can be obtained. The direction of shrinkage, combined with the almost instantaneous polymerization reaction of the light-cured resin composite, increases the polymerization contraction stresses to a level that exceeds the weak and slowly developing dentin bond.

This problem can be solved by taking advantage of the strain capacity of a given filling material: the results of tests for bonding strength indicate that materials with proper sealing ability do not necessarily show high bond strengths. They do, however, show an increased flexibility, or strain capacity, of the restorative system. Such a system can benefit from the application of an intermediate layer of a low-modulus material between tooth structures, corresponding with decreased marginal leakage scores. The importance of creating such an elasticity gradient down to the dentin-resin interface scale has been substantiated by nano-indentation measurements. Given these findings, glass-ionomer cements could be good materials to serve as such an intermediate layer, because they bond almost spontaneously to dentin, and on the condition that the strain capacity and , modulus of elasticity would render them suitable for such a system.

Characteristics of Glass-Ionomer Cements

Table 1-4 Physical properties of restorative filling materials

	Conventional Glass-Ionomer Cement	Resin-modified Glass-Ionomer Cement	Compomer	Resin Composite
Compressive strength, 1 day (MPa)	160 ~ 240	180 ~ 240	220 ~ 340	240 ~ 340
Flexural strength, 1 day (Mpa)	10 ~ 20	40 ~ 70	120 ~ 160	120 ~ 200
Fluoride release	+ +	+ +	+	−
Translucency	Poor	Good	Good	Good
Surface smoothness	−	− ~ ±	± ~ +	± ~ +
Radiopacity	+	+	+	+
Bond strength to bovine dentin, 1 day (MPa)				
To polished dentin	3 ~ 6	4 ~ 10	Does not bond	Does not bond
With treatment and/or	[illegible]	[illegible]	[illegible]	[illegible]

8. CHEMICAL AND BIOLOGICAL PROPERTIES OF GLASS-IONOMER CEMENTS:

Glass-ionomer cements are considered the most durable dental cements currently available, even though in an aqueous environment they are susceptible to hydrolytic degradation through erosion, ion release, and water sorption. Immediately after hardening, glass-ionomers are very sensitive to erosion because the matrix-forming ions are still soluble. When fully set, these cements release ions and absorb water in an aqueous environment. Conventional materials release sodium, fluoride, silica, and traces of calcium, whereas admixed amalgam alloy and cermets release additional ionic silver. The release of various ionic species from resin-modified glass- ionomers also has been confirmed.[4]

The water sorption phenomena from glass-ionomers have not been thoroughly investigated. From the early work of Wilson and Crisps it is known that the labile, loosely bound fraction of water in glass-ionomers reaches up to 5% by weight of the set cement. This fraction varies depending on the environmental conditions and results either in hygroscopic expansion or in shrinking and material crazing. These structural changes do not allow for a reliable gravimetric determination of water sorption employing and dry weighing methods. Nevertheless, in one study 3.8% water sorption was measured for a conventional product and considered as a clinical advantage because it exceeded the setting shrinkage of the material, although no values were provided for the latter.[4]

The introduction of visible light-cured resin-modified glass-ionomers was expected to provide protection against initial water sensitivity by the rapid formation of the polymer network, which would set up a barrier to water diffusion. However, it has been shown that these materials also absorb water because of the hydrophilic nature of their polymer networks, which incorporate 2-hydroxyethylmethacrylate (HEMA) or poly-HEMA and may adversely affect their properties. It seems that the retardation observed in the acid-base reaction rate of these products after the rapid formation of the photo polymerizable networking minimizes the benefits of any short-term shielding effect of the polymer matrix as opposed to the slow-developing polysalt matrix.

The solubility of glass-ionomers-the outcome of ion release and water uptake interactions has been investigated in solutions with acidic, neutral, or basic pH, utilizing immersion or jet erosion techniques. Most products were found to erode at a pH of less than 4, with the erosion rate depending mainly on the chemical composition of the cement and the setting status. Generally, polyacrylic acid-base cements are more erosion resistant than cements based on copolymers of acrylic and maleic acids. Silver cermet cements also demonstrate less erosion than do conventional materials. For resin-modified materials, higher erosion resistance was found due to the presence of the polymer network. Nevertheless, it has been shown that some products in this category, although they contain basic powder and polyacid components, are incapable of producing a polysalt matrix, an observation which puts in question their erosion resistance and clinical durability.

The dynamic equilibrium established between glass-ionomers and the oral environment substantially affects the reactivity of the materials through ion exchange processes, resulting in the release of ionic species of important biological activity. Among these, fluoride has attracted the most interest because of its documented ability to help prevent caries when added to oral health care products. It has been postulated that glass-ionomer restorations exert an anticariogenic effect on adjacent cavity walls in the event of primary or secondary caries attack. This effect has been attributed to the fluoride released which is absorbed by hard dental tissues, increasing their resistance to demineralization, enhancing remineralization reactions, and modifying carbohydrate metabolism of plaque. The complex mechanisms implemented in the development of the cariostatic effect of glass-ionomers in vitro, their in vivo relevance, and their clinical efficiency are discussed. The approach used is intended to facilitate understanding of the importance of the enormous number of in vitro findings compared to the limited amount of existing information for in vivo conditions.

Fluoride Release

The source of fluoride ions from glass-ionomer cements are the calcium fluoride (CaF_2)' strontium fluoride (SrF_2), lanthanull) fluoride (LaF_2)' sodium hexa- fiuoroaluminate (Na_3AlF_6)' and aluminum trifluoride (AlF_3) inclusions of the low- temperature glasses used to formulate the powder components. The primary role of these fluorides is to lower the glass fusion temperature during the manufacturing process, although they also improve handling properties and increase cement strength and translucency. During setting, the fluoride ions produced form strong soluble aluminofluoride complexes like AlF^{2+} and AlF^{2+}, which prevent premature gelation of poly ions by aluminum ions. In fully set cements, fluoride is located in the partially degraded glasses that form the glass core and in the polysalt matrix, primarily in the form of aluminum complexes.[45]

When a fully set glass-ionomer is exposed to neutral aqueous solutions, it absorbs water and releases ions such as sodium, silica, calcium, and fiuoride. Of the total amount of fluoride in the set cement, only a small fraction is available for release. This is not related to the total fluoride content of the cement, but depends on the amount of sodium that maintains cement electron neutrality after the fluoride release.Only the fluoride present in the matrix is available for elution at neutral conditions.

Mechanisms of fluoride release

Although many studies have reported a sustained release of fluoride from set glass-ionomer cements in distilled water over a long period of time. The mechanism of fluoride release is still not completely understood. It is generally accepted that two reactions are involved: a short-term reaction of high fluoride release corresponding to initial elution due to the postsetting maturation process, and a long-term reaction of low release attributed to equilibrium diffusion processes.

A systematic investigation of the fluoride release from a series of conventional and metal-reinforced glass-ionomer cements showed that the cumulative amount of fluoride released (Fc) in distilled water at 37°C as a function of *time* (t) corresponds to the following *equation:*

$$F c = (FI \times t) / (t + t_{1/2}) + (b \times \sqrt{t})$$

Where, FI is the maximum value of fluoride released during the short-term reaction period that occurs rapidly after specimen immersion in water and ceases after some days, *t1/2* is the half-life of the short-term reaction process, and b is a constant that expresses the measure of the driving force during the slow release period.[45]

The chemical composition and type of mixing were identified as the main factors affecting the kinetics of fluoride release. Amalgam alloy admixed cements were found to release amounts of fluoride higher than or equal to those of conventional glass-ionomers due to increased microporosity, which increases; the effective surface area for release. For silver cermet cements, in which silver particles are sintered to glass particles, the effective contact area between the glass particles and polyalkenoic acid is reduced, leading to a reduction in fluoride release, especially during the initial elution period. Resin-modified glass-ionomers release fluoride in distilled water at a range similar to those of conventional or metal-reinforced materials, but increased cumulative fluoride release or reduced short-term release rates have been noted in some products. The fact that the fluoride released from conventional products is mostly sodium fiuoride, along with the observation that this is not a critical salt for the formation of the polysalt matrix, explains the lack of anticipated weakening of the materials following fluoride release.

A significant increase in fluoride release is observed at low pH values, suggesting that an erosive mechanism is activated at these conditions from the preferential dissolution of the glass particles in the matrix. Another factor governing fluoride release is its concentration in the immersion solution. In the presence of an inverse fluoride concentration gradient, glass-ionomers may absorb fluoride from the environment and release it again under specific conditions. Thus, the concept of fluoride recharging old glass-ionomer fillings was introduced, in vitro evidence for which supports the theory that such interactions are feasible through an ion exchange process.[45]

Fluoride release and antibacterial activity of selected dental materials

A study was conducted to assess the fluoride ion release and antibacterial activities of the glassionomer cement Fuji IX and the compomer (composite modifi ed polyacid) Dyract AP.

Fluoride ion release was measured using direct potentiometry with an Orion fl uoride ion selective electrode. The measurement was carried out after 1, 4, 7, 14, 30, and 60 days of storage in phosphate buffer at pH 6.8. The antibacterial activity of the materials was evaluated against the bacteria *Streptococcus mutans ATCC 35668*, *Streptococcus salivarius ATCC 13419*,

Streptococcus sanguis ATCC 10556, and *Lactobacillus casei subsp. casei ATCC 393*. The agar diffusion test was applied. The material specimens were assessed twice: after setting and seven days later. Zones of bacterial growth inhibition were measured in millimeters after 24 hours.
The results of the study showed that both materials released ion fl uoride, with a higher emission of Fuji IX than Dyract AP. The highest level of emission was observed on the seventh day of the study in both materials. After 24 hours of bonding there was inhibition of bacterial growth by Fuji IX, whereas Dyract AP did not show similar activity. On the eighth day after polymerization, Dyract AP was significantly more active towards *Streptococcus sanguis* and *salivarius*.

Clinical relevance

The established fluoride releasing efficiency of glass-ionomers in aqueous solutions raised important questions as to the clinical relevance of this trait, and efforts were undertaken to investigate the fluoride release processes under conditions simulating the oral environment or in vivo. The first approach was to use artificial saliva. Comparative data on the fluoride release from the same brands of glass-ionomers in distilled water and artificial saliva revealed a reduction in the release when using the latter. When nonstimulated human saliva was used as an immersion medium, a significant reduction in fluoride release occurred which was mainly attributed to the adsorption of HPO_4^{2-} and saliva proteins onto material surfaces in the form of pellicle, inhibiting fluoride release.

The important question of whether the fluoride released from glass-ionomer cements is adequate to increase the fluoride concentration in saliva was addressed in several studies during the early 1990s. These studies provided evidence of elevated fluoride concentration in saliva for a period of a few weeks after glass-ionomer application, implying that these materials may be effective short-term intraoral fluoride releasing devices however, other in vivo experiments did not reach the same conclusion In some of these studies, the comparisons made among the fluoride release profiles in saliva were not reliable because lining materials were employed as restoratives.

Some conclusions may be drawn from the results of the fluoride release experiments. The experiments performed in distilled water or in any other artificial medium should be interpreted only on a material screening basis. Given that the actual amount of fluoride required to exert a cariostatic effect has not yet been determined, the varying levels of fluoride release should not be considered primary criteria for material selection, because very often materials with high fluoride release lack hydrolytic stability. It should be clearly stated that fluoride release is an ion exchange process, and ionic species are absorbed simultaneously from the environment to maintain diffusion equilibrium. In vivo the fluoride salivary levels may be increased after glass-ionomer application, but within a few weeks are reduced to baseline levels. From an experimental standpoint, the discrepancy in the way fluoride release data are presented is noteworthy. Cumulative fluoride values are usually given as a function of time in mg F^-, ppm F^-, mg F^- per unit volume of the cement, or mg F^- per surface area unit of the cement. The rationale for expressing the results in cumulative mode is seriously questioned because the experimental procedure for measuring fluoride release involves an open system, in which partial or complete replacement of the immersion liquid occurs at specific time intervals. It should be stated that the fiuoride selective electrode measurements represent the maximum amount of ionizable fluoride available in the solution and not the actual ionized fraction, due to the addition of the total ionic strength adjustment buffer solution. In the case of fluoride units, elution is considered a surface phenomenon and the results should be expressed in mass per unit of total specimen surface area to allow for direct comparisons among materials.

Fluoride Uptake

Several in vitro studies have shown that substantial amounts of fluoride released from glass-ionomer restorations are taken up by sound enamel and dentin cavity walls this release also has been confirmed by in vivo studies. However, the results presented should be interpreted with caution, because in some approaches where electron probe microanalysis was employed to investigate the elemental composition at interfaces between a glass-ionomer and enamel or dentin, no secondary or backscattered electron images of the analyzed regions were provided. The distributions of calcium and silica used in these studies to determine the exact position of the edge of the cavity wall lack accurate spatial resolution, especially if the high calcium concentration of the glass-ionomers used (which further complicates signal interpretation) is considered. Under these conditions it is possible that morphologic irregularities at the interface could be misinterpreted as elemental diffusion gradients, denoting selective uptake.[49]

Another important problem when studying the interfaces of glass ionomers under the high-vacuum, high-energy incident probes required for this type of analysis is the excessive dehydration of the cements and the resulting dimensional changes. A common artifact is cracking and debonding of the material from hard tissues. In such cases residual small glass-ionomer particles attached to enamel or dentin could be considered evidence of elemental diffusion. Consequently, a high-resolution image of the interface is of critical importance for elemental characterization at this region.

The limitations of establishing the real interface in characterizing elemental gradients also apply to more sophisticated techniques. For example, a submicron resolution in depth proiling during secondary ion mass spectrometry (SIMS) measurements may lack precision in determining interfacial gradients on dentin surfaces polished with 600-grit SiC paper, which creates a mean roughness at a micron scale, implicating features. Furthermore, surface contamination during sectioning or polishing may comprise a significant source of error, especially when highly sensitive surface analysis techniques are used.

The problems encountered in such complex analytical situations have been described by Duschner et al. These authors analyzed the enamel cavity walls of teeth restored with a glass-ionomer and stored in sterile filtered saliva for 6 weeks, using complementary advanced micro-analytical techniques such as small-area photoelectron spectroscopy, laser ablation mass spectrometry, and confocal laser scanning microscopy. This multi-technique characterization confirmed that fluoride did not migrate into the enamel of the cavity wall. However, SIMS line scan experiments performed at glass-ionomer-dentin interfaces have clearly demonstrated fluoride uptake in dentin of 100 to 300 μm from the interface, hich overwhelms any doubts regarding interfacial interferences. Dentin pre-treatment with acid etching substantially modifies dentin fluoride uptake by altering tissue permeability.[49]

An alternative experiment performed in vivo measured the amount of fluoride absorbed by the uppermost 10μm of enamel bonded to a glass-ionomer cement at sequential micron intervals, using the biopsy technique after mechanical removal of the cement. However, no information was given on the efficiency of the removal method to minimize interferences from residual glass-ionomer particles, a parameter for acknowledged as a possible source of error.

Based on all of these results, it is obvious that there is still no sound evidence to support fluoride diffusion from glass-ionomer restorations to the bonded enamel walls. In vivo experiments are needed to verify the in vitro findings for dentin walls. An interesting mode of fluoride uptake concerned enamel or cementum surfaces adjacent to, but not in contact with, the margins of glass-ionomer restorations. In vitro studies employing this approach have demonstrated increased fluoride concentration at these regions, but the effect was not documented in vivo.

The status of the fluoride absorbed by hard dental tissues bonded to glass ionomers is not known. The aspects concerning fluoroapatite, calcium fluoride, or nonspecifically absorbed fluoride formation are well documented in the field of topically applied fluoride agents and dentifrices, but not for glass-ionomer cements. For the latter, an assumption is made that the reactivity of the fluoride released is similar to that found in oral health care products. It is reasonable to expect that the initial low pH of glass-ionomers may induce dissolution of the adjacent apatite and redeposition of calcium salts incorporating fluoride, which is initially released at high rates. Evidence to support such an interaction has been presented in only one in vitro study, where fluoridated carbonoapatite was identified at the interface between a conventional glass-ionomer restorative and cavity walls. Apparently these interactions take place at the demineralization front and not at sites distant from the interface. It is interesting to note that the only fluorinated compound identified in vitro in bulk tissue was located on dentin. Dentin demonstrates greater fluoride uptake than enamel due to the former's greater porosity, increased water content, smaller crystalline size, and presence of the organic phase (which seems to be an important factor in fluoride uptake procedures). It has been shown that the organic components of dentin, such as collagen and non-collagenous proteins, take up significantly higher amounts of fluoride released from glass-ionomers than do the inorganic components and also have a high binding capacity. This fraction of fluoride is being believed to be involved in dentin mineralization procedures. Unfortunately, no further information exists on the state of fluoride at glass-ionomer dentin interfaces.[50]

The concentration of fluoride in plaque, the physical in vivo barrier to fluoride in evolution from glass-ionomers has been the subject of many studies during the last decade. In situ experiments have shown high levels of fluoride in plaque growing adjacent to glass-ionomer restorations, while in vivo experiments have demonstrated that the fluoride content was greatly increased in plaque adjacent to glass-ionomers even 4 weeks after their application. However, aged glass- ionomer specimens placed intraorally were found to accumulate more plaque with reduced fluoride content relative to fresh material. Still, the plaque fluoride content was higher than that of a resin composite control. These findings support the theory that plaque developed on glass-ionomer restorations may act as a fluoride pool in the microenvironment of the restoration.[51]

A critical point in understanding the role of the fluoride acquired in pellicle and plaque adjacent to glass-ionomer cements in the interfacial availability of the fluoride is to identify its binding states in these integuments. So far, no studies have been published in this area. However, from the total amount of fluoride found in dental plaque, less than 1% is in an ionized state, a fraction is in the form of calcium phosphate precipitates which nay be released at low pH, and the vast majority is strongly bound to macro-molecules and bacteria. Thus, the concept that dental plaque may act as a fluoride reservoir for adjacent hard dental tissues during remineralization periods may apply only to fully fluoride saturated plaque, if such conditions can be established intraorally. The main reason is that as pH rises during remineralization, urea and amine production from plaque is increased, reaching optimum values at about pH 5.59 These basic components demonstrate high chemical affinity to any fluoride in the region, forming stable compounds. Regarding the potential of in vivo recharging of aged glass-ionomers, preliminary results indicate that recharging had no beneficial effect on the fluoride concentration of adjacent plaque.[51]

The antibacterial properties of glass-ionomers documented in vitro failed to inhibit plaque growth on their surfaces in vivo. However, the composition of the plaque that accumulated on glass-ionomers showed a reduction in the proportion of *mutans streptococci.* Furthermore, observations that this proportion increased as glass-ionomer restorations aged implies that the short-term reaction of fluoride release is closely associated with the microbial inhibition. These effects found to be limited to the vicinity of local environment without affecting the plaque on adjacent teeth.[52]

The relationship between fluoride content and fluoride release for glass-ionomer cements is not well understood. A study was done to determine the fluoride concentrations at the surfaces of glass-ionomer materials with respect to different storage media and different pH environments; to examine the recharge ability of the materials after NaF immersion; and to assess the morphological changes at the material surfaces using scanning electron microscope and energy dispersive spectroscopic techniques (SEM/EDS).Five glass-ionomer materials, Fuji Triage (FT), Fuji II LC (FII), Fuji VIII (FVIII), Fuji IX GP(FIX), and Ketac N100 (KN), were analyzed in this study. Resin-based fluoride releasing material Helioseal F (HSF) was used as a comparison material. The sample consisted of 120 cured cement disks (n = 20 disks of each tested material, 10 × 1.5 mm). Five disks of each material were stored in 4 different storage media (I- saline, II- acidic solution ph = 2.5, III- acid solution ph = 5.5, IV- NaF solution (c = 500/106). After 7 days, two disks of each material were transferred from media I, II and III to the NaF solution for 3 min. EDS analysis was conducted in 3 randomly selected spots of each experimental disk. SEM was used to determine morphological characteristics of the material surface. Differences between the experimental groups have been analyzed using Student's t-test with the level of significance set at $p < 0.001$.

FT showed the highest fluoride content at the surface of the material. The lowest amounts of fluoride ions were detected at the surfaces of the FT disks stored at low pH environments, and this difference was statistically significant ($p < 0.001$). Glass-ionomers showed significantly higher fluoride concentrations when compared to the HSF ($p < 0.001$). After immersion in the NaF solution, fluoride concentrations at the surfaces of the disks increased when compared with previous storage media (FT>FVIII>KN>FII>FIX). SEM analysis of the surface morphology revealed numerous voids, cracks and microporosities in all experimental groups, except for KN and HSF. More homogenous material structure with more discrete cracks was observed in samples stored at neutral pH environment, compared to disks stored in acidic solutions. The tested materials could be considered as promising dental materials with potential prophylactic characteristics due to their relatively high fluoride content, but also the ability to extensively reabsorb fluoride ions, especially in acidic environments.

Remineralization of Adjacent Hard Tissues

The fluoride uptake of hard dental tissues adjacent to glass-ionomer materials has been considered a fundamental factor for inhibition of secondary caries attack. Today, however, it is generally accepted that fluoride uptake alone does not necessarily imply caries reduction susceptibility. The determining factor is the secondary mobility of fluoride absorbed by the tissues, which reflects the ability of the fluoridated compounds formed to establish a solution equilibrium at the interface during demineralization and remineralization cycles.

In vitro studies

To evaluate the performance of the fluoride released from glass-ionomer restorations under simulated conditions of secondary caries attack, a series of artificial caries experiments were conducted and showed that the frequency and extent of outer and wall lesions was reduced around glass-ionomer restorations in vitro. The reduction in the extent of the outer lesion, which is considered to resemble primary caries, was attributed to the diffusion of fluoride ions through the artificial caries medium, whereas the reduction in the depth of the wall lesion was attributed to the low solubility of the cavity walls to the hydrogen ion diffusion gradient set at the interface, due to fluoride release and uptake procedures.Limited information is available on the composition of the artificial caries lesions. Studies of artificial lesions on dentin walls in contact with glass-ionomers showed that the levels of calcium and phosphorous in lesion bodies were decreased relative to the organic component; in inhibited zones these levels were similar to those in sound dentin, but the level of fluoride was significantly higher.

In several in vitro studies, demineralization and remineralization cycles were performed to better simulate intraoral pH fluctuations. These studies documented that glass-ionomers prevent demineralization of adjacent enamel and hyper mineralize dentin walls through a, mechanism possibly associated with the formation of calcium fluoride deposits. These findings were consistently obtained from fresh glass-ionomer restorations, but no similar effects were documented for aged specimens. The clinical relevance of these findings has not been verified. The absence of pellicle, plaque, and bacteria and the strong acidic environment used in vitro to mimic acid production by bacteria intraorally, invalidate the extrapolation of the in vitro findings to in vivo conditions. Direct comparison is not even feasible between the in vitro reported studies because the composition of the acidified gels, the demineralizing or remineralizing solutions used, the pH, and the duration of the testing periods vary greatly.

In vivo studies

The extensive use of in vitro models to simulate the in vivo situation and the criticism of such simplified approaches established the need for controlled studies of fluoride releasing materials in the oral environment. The first approach was to design in situ experiments. Several models were developed for the study of the interfaces of enamel or dentin with fluoride releasing materials placed in partial dentures or other removable appliances worn intraorally for periods of 1 to 3 months. These models incorporated assessment of several variables, such as the presence of a standardized interfacial gap between the restoration and tissues, the presence of an artificial carious lesion, or the simulation of high cariogenic challenge by immersing the specimens in sucrose solution at specific time intervals. The results confirmed the beneficial effects of fluoride release to the adjacent tissues for the time periods tested. Of particular importance was the finding that, in cases of interfacial discontinuities in the form of gaps, the amount of fluoride released into the liquid in the gap is of much greater importance than the amount of fluoride taken up by tissues.

A modification of the standardized gap model also has been used for in vivo assessment of the enamel anticariogenic potential of glass-ionomers for orthodontic band cementation. The experimental design included the development of a standardized microspace between cemented bands and enamel to accumulate plaque. Four weeks after band cementation, the mineral content of the lesion found around glass-ionomer cements was significantly higher than that around a nonfluoride containing phosphate cement used as a control. This design, however, did not take into account the strong initial acidic challenge of a setting phosphate cement to the micro- space; the pH of phosphate cements remains below 5 even 24 hours after setting, while the corresponding values for glass-ionomers range from 5.5 to 6.5. Thus it is not known whether the initial acidic environment created around the phosphate cement affected the total mineral loss observed.

A common finding in the in vivo studies concerning the anticariogenic properties of glass-ionomers is that the experimental period is limited to the first few weeks after placement of the restorations. It is well established that during this period, glass-ionomers exert the highest fluoride release rate and the strongest antibacterial activity. The long-term performance of the cariostatic properties of glass-ionomer cements has not been systematically investigated, and the information currently available is limited to clinical studies reporting secondary caries incidence with all the associated diagnostic limitations.

Several clinical studies have documented a low incidence of secondary caries adjacent to glass-ionomer restorations. However, two recently published articles, based on surveys of the reasons for restoration replacement in general dental practice, reported relatively high incidences of secondary caries in relation to glass-ionomer restoration failures. These findings forced the authors to emphasize the urgent need for further studies to confirm the anticariogenic effect in vivo.

To investigate the anticariogenic efficiency of glass-ionomers over a longer period, a study was designed introducing an artificial gap model in vivo and correlating the results with the same model under artificial caries attack. Briefly, at the mid-buccal area of sound premolars to be extracted for orthodontic reasons, paired Class V cavities limited to enamel were prepared in each patient. Lesions were filled with a conventional glass-ionomer and a non-fluoride containing light-cured resin composite on contralateral sides after placing thick metal spacers at the incisal walls of the cavities to create artificial gaps. The incisal walls received no conditioning or priming treatments. After setting, the spacers were removed and, after 6 months, the teeth were extracted, sectioned, and studied under polarized light. The same procedure was used to restore cavities prepared at the buccal area of sound premolars extracted for orthodontic reasons, which were then subjected to an artificial caries experiment using an acidified gel (pH 4) for 4 weeks.

The in vitro findings of the study confirmed the cariostatic effect of glass- ionomers in gap-free regions, as shown in many previous studies, as well as its beneficial role in the presence of interfacial gaps. However, the in vivo findings demonstrated a different lesion pattern. No lesions were observed at gap-free restorations. In the presence of artificial gaps, the area of lesions adjacent to the glass-ionomer was greater than that adjacent to the resin composite. The depth of the enamel wall lesion, the length of the superficial mineralized enamel, and the extent of the underlying demineralized region were increased in cavities restored with glass-ionomer. These preliminary results show that some glass-ionomers may not exert an efficient anticariogenic effect at adjacent enamel walls in vivo in the presence of an interfacial gap. They also highlight the role of gap-free restorations in reducing secondary caries incidence.

Optimization of the adhesive and sealing properties of glass-ionomer cements may provide protection against secondary caries, until the expected anticariogenic activity of the fluoride released is established in well-defined in vivo models and controlled clinical studies. Unfortunately, such an effect has not yet been fully documented.

Chemical exchange between glass-ionomer restorations and residual carious dentine in permanent molars[58]

A study was done to evaluate the remineralization of carious dentine following the restoration of an extensive lesion in a permanent molar with a high strength glass-ionomer cement (GIC). Thirteen first permanent molars, which were scheduled for extraction because of the presence of extensive caries lesions, were selected for this study. They were first restored, according to the ART technique, using encapsulated Fuji IXGP, which contains a strontium glass rather than the traditional calcium glass. The cavities were prepared with a clean enamel margin and minimal removal of the carious dentine around the walls. After a period of 1–3 months they were harvested and subsequently sectioned and examined using an electron probe microanalysis (EPMA) and scanning electronmicroscopy (SEM).

EPMA demonstrated that both fluorine and strontium ions had penetrated deep into the underlying demineralized dentine. The only possible source of these ions was the GIC restoration. The pattern of penetration of the fluorine and strontium ions into the dentine was consistent with a remineralization process.

Effects of a glass-ionomer cement on the remineralization of occlusal caries – an *in situ* study

This work evaluated the remineralization of demineralized enamel of pits and fissures of human third molars sealed with a glass ionomer cement (Fuji IX, GC Corporation - Japan) or with a Bis-GMA sealant (Delton -Dentsply). Ten volunteers participated in this *in situ* study that consisted of two thirty-day periods using intra-oral devices, with a week's interval in between. Four experimental treatment procedures and one control were randomly assigned to the volunteers' specimens: Group I, no treatment, control; Group II, artificial caries process; Group III, same treatment as Group II, but sealed with Delton (Dentsply); Group IV, same treatment as Group II, but sealed with Fuji IX (GC Corporation - Japan); Group V, same treatment as Group II and no sealing. Groups I and II were not submitted to the oral environment and served as controls. After a period of 30 days in the oral environment, the specimens were removed from the devices, embedded in acrylic resin, ground flat and polished. Then, Knoop hardness tests were performed, with a 25 g static load applied for 15 seconds. The measurements were made from the base of the fissure up to an opening of 600 μm, pre-established between the inclines of the cusps. Three indentations were then made, located at 25, 75, and 125 μm in depth from the outer enamel margin and 100 μm apart from each other (Micromet 2003). The Brieger F and Bonferroni's tests were applied to the measurements. It was concluded that sealing with the glass ionomer cement Fuji IX was capable of making the enamel of pits and fissures more resistant by increasing the value of Knoop hardness.

9. BIOCOMPATIBILITY OF GLASS-IONOMER CEMENTS

Glass-ionomer cements seem to be beneficial from a clinical point of view because of their continuous release of fluoride which reduces the rate of a secondary caries both in filled teeth and on the enamel surfaces of adjacent teeth. Fewer microorganisms are found in remaining carious dentin subjacent to glass-ionomer restorations, and there is actually a fluoride uptake in human dentin. Another great advantage of glass-ionomers is the continuous uptake of fluoride, which may greatly extend the beneficial effects of these materials.[57]

The first group of glass-ionomers on the market had a low pH during the initial setting period and therefore had adverse effects on pulpal tissues when the residual dentin was thin. Although improvements have been made to these materials, especially with the addition of resins, there are still some questions with respect to the biocompatibility of glass-ionomer cements.

Biocompatibility and Cytotoxicity of Dental Biomaterials

It is well documented that some dental biomaterials are harmful and others are not. Months or years after cavities are created and filled with cements or resins, the pulp may react and undergo degeneration. When oxyphosphate cements containing orthophosphoric acid were used for luting or filling, the reaction was acute and painful; pulp necrosis sometimes followed pulpitis. With other biomaterials the reaction was gradual and almost silent, but pulp degeneration still occurred. In many cases, no reaction was observed, and dentin deposition in the pulp chamber together with a living pulp surviving tissue was considered as a success.

Even with the development of new materials such as adhesive and resin composites, glass-ionomer cements, and mixtures of glass-ionomer and resin composite, there are still reactions. However, they are less frequent and those that occur escape the attention of clinicians, with asymptomatic pulp apoptosis.

There is no legal requirement for a systematic study of pulp status after the introduction of new dental biomaterials. Therefore, the continuous influx of new materials to the market does not allow in vivo evaluations and in vitro tests of the biocompatibility or toxicity of these materials. The evolution of dental products is so rapid that as soon a new material is put in the market, it is outdated, with another version appearing within weeks or months and claiming to be extensively improved. As a consequence, no systematic studies are carried out on the pathology induced by recent adhesives, composites, or glass ionomers.

Bergenholtz has shown that the presence of bacteria between the cavity surface and the restorative material is responsible for pulp reaction. In this context, a clear relationship was drawn between the presence of bacteria and the diffusion of exotoxins in dental tubules toward the pulp. This phenomenon was especially true for many products available in the 1980s. At that time, there was always a crevice between the wall of the cavity and the filling. Some contraction of the filling was due to dehydration during preparation of samples, and shrinkage was enhanced by the high vacuum used when samples were observed with scanning electron microscopy (SEM). It is widely accepted that the gap between the biomaterial and dental tissue was about 10 to 25μm, a width which allowed hundreds of microorganisms to penetrate the interface simultaneously.

New adhesives have since been developed and, from the literature, it is clear that no gaps exist between fillings and cavity walls that might be colonized by bacteria. The formation of a hybrid layer also prohibits the formation of such gaps, Therefore, two possibilities exist: (1) bacteria located at the resin-dentin interface are responsible for the harmful reactions and the problem should be solved by improving the adhesives and biomaterials, or (2) the diffusion of uncontrolled components of the bio- materials induces pulp alterations. It may be derived from this that many biological problems still need to be solved to avoid pulp reactions from dental biomaterials.[59]

Pulp Biology

The embryonic pulp develops together with the dental lamina and enamel organ in the first branchial arch. In mammals early emigrating midbrain crest cells migrate to the dental mesenchyma. These cells appear in the condensing mesenchyme and in the dental papilla. After a fixed number of mitotic divisions, they appear at the surface of the embryonic pulp either as postmitotic odontoblasts, which differentiate, polarize, and acquire all the biological properties of dentin-forming cells, or as daughter cells that have no direct contact to the basement membrane, or Hohl layer. The participation of cells originating from the para-axial mesenchyme has still not been determined, but it is highly probable that some pulp components are not of neural crest origin. Cells migrate from the dental sac and adjacent mesenchyma and remain in the central part of the pulp. In this context, the sprouting of endothelial cells and axon growth during pulp morphogenesis leads to the development of vascularization and innervation.

After the onset of tooth formation, any replacement of postmitotic odontoblasts can damage or destroy these cells. Cells from the Hohl layer have the same embryonic origin as the odontoblasts; therefore, it can be hypothesized that they have the potential to differentiate and become replacement cells acting as odontoblasts. In adult pulp, no cell population can differentiate, polarize, and act as second-generation odontoblasts, but some precursor cells contribute to the deposition of reparative dentin.

Cell differentiation in adult pulp

Some undifferentiated cells located in the central pulp-called mesenchymal stem cells, pericytes, endothelial cells, or fibro blasts-keep the potential for differentiation and become mitotic. In the case of experimental pulp capping, after a first mitosis, they migrate toward a wounded zone and a second mitosis occurs. The daughter cells then differentiate into replacement cells capable of producing a mineralized layer of what seems to be osteodentin.

Vascularization and innervation both play essential roles in pulp biology, including the provision of nutrients to the tissue. In addition, pulp cells have their own specificity's.

Specialized pulp cells

Pulp fibroblasts, or pulpoblasts, exhibit specific differences from other cells. They are never isolated but are linked one to another by intercellular (desmosome-like and gap) junctions. This relationship implies a continuity in the cell network inside the pulp, from the center where they emerge and differentiate toward the outer pulp beneath the Hohl layer and the odontoblasts.

It is interesting to note that mitosis is hardly detected in adult pulp for unknown reasons. It is hardly conceivable that mitotic cells can be present during the whole life of the tooth as neurons are. In noncarious teeth, the percentage of cells bearing the proliferating cell nuclear antigen is low compared with cells derived from periodontal ligament, bone stroma, and muscular tissue. There is increased labeling only in cases of advanced caries. Labeling with the silver-binding nucleolar organizer region (AgNOR) stain provides the same type of information. In addition, it has been shown that there is no difference between the coronal and radicular areas of the pulp in this respect. They both display low labeling, except in response to caries.

There is a population of immuno competent cells in normal dental pulp. Dendritic cells, T lymphocytes, and macrophages have been identified in rat incisor. The hypothesis that these cells are present in case of aggression is unacceptable. In an investigation carried out on the pulp of essential fatty acid-deficient (EFAD) rats, cell density in EFAD rats was double that in control rats. One possible explanation of this phenomenon may be that the influence of the deficiency on arachidonic metabolism (less than half the value found in control rats) interferes with the synthesis of prostaglandins and leukotriens. In such circumstances, deregulation of apoptosis, a phenomenon known to be prostaglandin dependent and involved in the control of cell number, can lead to the increase in density that was noted. When three methods- TUNEL staining, anti-transglutaminase, and characteristic morphology-were used to identify apoptotic cells, most pulp cells did not react, with the exception of a few located in the outer pulp beneath the Hohl layer and odontoblasts.

All together, the distribution and labeling of cells show that undifferentiated cells appear in the central pulp. As soon as they differentiate into pulpoblasts, they establish strong links due to the presence of functional complexes and form a dense network. Cells are further transported subjacent to odontoblasts, where immunocompetent cells act as killers to control the cell population. Cells move toward the outer pulp where killer cells such as dendritic cells, lymphocytes, and cells expressing Class II antigen are present. As is usual in apoptosis, intercellular junctions are disrupted. Individual cells are subjected to specific chromatin changes in the nuclei and disintegrate. Residual apoptotic bodies are easily observed in the pulp. Cell remnants are destroyed by macrophages. If this interpretation is correct, it implies that immunocompetent cells are not involved in normal pulp defense processes, nor in rescuing the pulp in case of aggression. However, these cells are implicated in the control of pulp cell populations. In this context, the mechanisms of cytotoxicity can be considered the deregulation of a normal cell control mechanism.

Results of in vivo studies are difficult to compare because of the many parameters involved, including legal restrictions and extrapolation from young, healthy teeth to carious, older teeth and from animal models to human specimens. Thus, research must be carried out using in vitro systems to study biological reactions.

Pulp cells in culture

When pulp from neonatal mice with intact odontoblasts was isografted to spleen, tubular dentin was produced. In contrast, ectomesenchymal cells of dental papilla transplanted in isogenic mouse spleen produced only osteodentin-like material and orthodentin. Assuming that the culture model is representative of the exposed pulp in vivo, cells were cultured from human pulp explants. These specimens were different from fibroblast- like cells. At the beginning, the young cells were round or elongated with thin spinous processes, were highly mobile, and contained numerous lipid vesicles as evidenced with Oil Red O stain under a light microscope and by osmiumimidazole electron-dense lipid droplets seen on ultrathin sections under an electron microscope. These lipids probably originated from pinocytotic activity because no active synthesis was revealed by 1-[^{14}C] palmitic acid incorporation. It is known that marrow cells can differentiate, under some culture conditions, into adipocytes that convert along the osteogenic pathway. cells display strong alkaline phosphate staining and are able to form mineralized nodules.[23] This formation of nodules can be used as a model to study either pathologic pulp mineralizations or the formation of what has been called *reparative dentin*· This type of cell culture has been widely used for in vitro investigations on the biocompatibility of dental biomaterials, including glass-ionomer cements.

In Vivo Studies an Humans and Animals

The original composition of glass-ionomer powders was based on a formulation of silicon dioxide, aluminum oxide, calcium, fluoride, aluminum phosphate, and sodium hexafluoroaluminate. This allowed a possible toxic reaction from aluminum. Other components, such as fluoride, corundum, strontium, barium, lanthanum, zinc oxide, and zirconium oxide, are now used to increase opacity. Some glass-ionomers use a copolymer of acrylic acid to control the viscosity of the polyacrylic acid. Some of these acids are or not biocompatible. Stronger glass-ion- piomer cements are produced by the addition of 2-hydroxyethylmethacrylate (HEMA), which is capable of free radical polymerization. Developments in the re formulation of resin-modified glass-ionomers also have enhanced their properties and are widely used. Metal particles, fibers, or powders in cermet cements have significantly improved resistance to abrasion. This adds another parameter to the potential cytotoxicity of glass-ionomers. Thus, three groups of components of glass-ionomer cements can induce adverse reactions: the glass-ionomer itself, metals that are added to the cement and non polymerized resin components. Each of these components presents its own problems and may contribute to adverse reactions.

Tissue reactions can be ranked from moderate to severe, although in some reports pulp reactions have been evaluated as none, slight, moderate, severe. Moderate responses exhibit a predominant population of lymphocytes, and sometimes giant cells and macrophages; capillary proliferation; and fibroblasts and fibrocytes. Severe responses are characterized by a mixture of granulocytes and lymphocytes, predominant capillary proliferation, and a large number of giant cells and macrophages.

The initial acidity of glass-ionomer cements (close to pH 2 at 5 minutes after placement and pH 3 at 10 minutes) may contribute to pulp reaction. This was the case for the first generation of glass-ionomers, especially when they were used as luting agents. Pameijer and Stanley observed pulpal abscesses and intense hemorrhage when a glass-ionomer was used under continuous pressure and the remaining dentin thickness was 0.5 mm or less. This was the case when the study involved a full crown preparation. Some pulpal action, including abscesses and haemorrhage, persisted even after 60 days. Stanley concluded that when remaining dentin thickness is less than 1 mm, there is a need for pulpal protection before glass-ionomer cements used.[63]

In cell culture, initial tests indicate that traditional glass-ionomer cements are cytotoxic, but no adverse response is found with light-cured glass-ionomers. Animal experiments have shown that direct contact of cements with pulp tissues causes necrosis and should be avoided. Human studies of glass-ionomer, restorations in Class I sites in premolars have shown inflammation in 5% of the pulps. Correlation between pulpal inflammation and bacterial microleakage was found by Browne et.al. This group concluded that the potential chemical inflammation was of only minor importance. Sensitivity after Class III and Class V restorations was minimal with glass-ionomer fillings. When Class V cavities were prepared in 170 adult dog teeth and 20 Class I cavities in human teeth, it was concluded that a combination of glass-ionomer and light-cured composite was superior to the composite restoration alone because fewer microorganisms were present with the former. No correlation was found between pathologic results and remaining dental thickness, but there was a correlation between bacteria and inflammation.

The present authors carried out human studies several years ago following Class V preparations on premolars of 12 to 14 year old patients. Teeth were prepared and filled with a light-cured glass-ionomer cement that is no longer commercially available. After 8 days, 1 month, or 3 months they were extracted and treated according to the Recommended standard Practices for Biological Evaluation of Dental Biomaterials (ISO Technical Report 7405, 1984) and further processed for examination by light microscope. The results of pulpal reaction were ranked from slight to moderate after 1 month. However, after 3 months the pulp in 8 of 10 teeth was seriously damaged. Large areas in the pulp had been destroyed, but the odontoblast layer had not. At the time, the authors were unfamiliar with apoptotic degeneration of tissues and were unable to provide a clear-cut explanation of the results. Because odontoblasts are located adjacent to the dentinal tubules, it seemed logical that reactions would occur in this layer first and subsequently in the pulp. However, it is now well documented that apoptosis occurs more often in cells undergoing mitosis than in postmitotic cells. Thus, the fact that odontoblasts are postmitotic cells and that pulp cells keep this potential property may be relevant. The reactions seen in this study were not limited to light cured glass-ionomer cements. Less dramatic phenomena occurred with some adhesives and resins.

The authors obtained different results with another light-cured glass-ionomer (Fuji II LC). The biocompatibility of this glass-ionomer cement was good, most teeth displaying reactions ranking from none to moderate. When this cement was used to restore Class V cavities in sound dentin, tubular orthodentin was deposited adjacent to a marked calciotraumatic line. This finding is worth noting because in most cases, after the placement of adhesive, resin, or cement fillings, reparative dentin is of the osteo-dentin type, often without tubules and comprising cell inclusions within the mineralized tissue. Despite the specificity of the model and the small size of the animals, the authors next developed a rat model. Rats were anesthetized intraperitoneally with 6% chloral. After electosurgery of the gingiva and using a stereoscopic microscope at magnification, two cavities were prepared on the mesial aspect of each of the maxillary molars in 1 to 2 seconds with a high-speed contra-angle handpiece working at 120,000 rpm. Round cavities were prepared through half the thickness of the dentin. The tungsten carbide bur (0.05 ISO) was changed after every fourth cavity. No water-cooling was used; cavities were rinsed with a wet cotton pellet and dried with a gentle blast of air. Sixteen cavities were filled with a light-cured glass-ionomer, five with Compoglass, and eight with Dyract. As controls, cavities with no retention were left unfilled. After demineralization of block sections of the teeth, 7μm-thick sections were stained with Masson's, hematoxylin-eosin, and Brown and Brenn for bacterial demonstration.

In most cases, no adverse pulp reaction was seen, and the worst reactions that did occur were moderate. Results for the glass-ionomers were compared to those for two adhesives and two resin composites. In sections prepared from rats allowed to survive 8 days following the placement of the filling material, a severe reaction was seen in each section of the 6 teeth treated with one adhesive.

TUNEL labeling detected apoptosis in a group of cells in the zone connected with the tubules emerging from the lower cervix. Odonto- blasts were not damaged. Osteodentin was seen in both experimental and control specimens. No clear relationship could be established between the presence of bacteria and the adverse reactions. In some cases, a thin red layer was present at the interface between the biomaterial and the cavity wall. In other cases, microorganisms were seen in the dentinal tubules. Brown and Brenn stained slides revealed that, in this animal model, bacteria were not present when the cavity was left unfilled. This is probably due to the fact that food intake has a self-cleaning effect on the surface of the open cavity. In contrast, in cavities filled with either glass-ionomers or resin composites, bacteria were present at the filling-dentin interface and, in many cases, inside the lumen. This finding limits the conclusions that can be reached with this model, dealing with the specificity of the animal model versus actual human clinical studies. However, in most cases using this model, glass-ionomer cements were found to be biocompatible.

In Vitro Studies

Due to the lack of confidence in animal models and to the complexity of in vivo or clinical studies, in vitro approaches have been proposed. There are a few reports on the cytotoxicity and components of conventional and light-cured glass- ionomer cements. Imazato et al showed that VitreBond lining cement is extremely cytotoxic, while the toxicity of Fuji Lining LC and Ketac Bond is negligible. This investigation was carried out on L-929 mouse fibroblasts. According to the findings, the concentration of zinc in the cement seems to affect the degree of toxicity, whereas concentrations of silicon, aluminum, calcium, and strontium do not. Although the eluate for VitreBond contained about 6.9 times the HEMA concentration of Fuji Lining LC, the implication of this molecule in cytotoxicity is still uncertain. Using MTT assay, Kan et al detected minimal reduction in percentage absorbance values for the four materials evaluated. Resin composite and Fuji II LC eluate exhibited close to 100% cell growth 1 day after extraction, whereas with conventional glass-ionomer and Vitremer the percentage of control was 85.7 and 73.6, respectively. The conclusion was that fluoride release did not account for the cytotoxicity observed. From this study and others it can be concluded that the cytotoxicity of glass-ionomer cements is not due to fluoride release, but to unidentified toxic components diffusing into the culture medium or components of resins.

On a clone of L-929 mouse fibroblasts, Chem-Fil, Ketac-Fil, and Ketac-silver gave excellent results in percentage of control growth with the MTT test, whereas the percentage of cell growth for VitreBond was low. Results obtained following surgical implantation into bone did not conflict with the results from direct cell contact.

In another experiment, five glass-ionomer cements were put in direct contact with cultured human osteoblastic cells. The plating efficiency, adhesion, osteocalcin production, and morphology of the cells were tested. The results indicated that four of the five cements (Ketac-Fil Aplicap, Fuji II, Fuji II LC, and Ionocem Ionocap) are biocompatible when they are put in contact with this biological material, whereas Vitremer exhibits a marked toxicity toward the cells. {The key component thought to be released from RMGIC is HEMA.HEMA when released from it can diffuse through dentin and this effects the pulp.

This has been studied in detail by Hamid and Hum [65]where they used extracted molars wih degrees of caries and HEMA was supplied in a bonding resin and diffusion of HEMA was studied usin g high performance liquid chromatography.These experiments showed two things [65]

1. Dentin under all conditions of caries severity,including caries free,allowed HEMA to diffuse through due to its hydrophilicity and low molecular weight, thus reaching dental pulp cells

2. Severely carious teeth showed a markedly higher rate of diffusion than teeth with either mild or moderate caries.

3. Decreasing thickness of dentin markedly increased the rate of diffusion of HEMA towards the pulp.}

Oliva et al attributed the adverse reaction to the leaching of HEMA from the cement. The addition of pure HEMA at the same concentration found by protonic magnetic resonance analysis. The adverse reaction was attributed by these authors to the leaching of HEMA. The concentration of HEMA was evaluated by protonic magnetic resonance analysis. When pure HEMA was added to the culture medium at the same concentration, the same toxic effects were observed. This conclusion corroborates the assumption that unpolymerized and leachable resin components, such as Bis-GMA, urethane dimethacrylate (UDMA), triethylene glycol dimethacrylate (TEGDMA), and Bis-phenol A, have major cytotoxic effects. These monomeric resin components are not only toxic to fibroblasts in culture but can evoke immunosuppression or immunostimulation on mitogen-driven proliferation of purified lymphocytes

In vitro studies were carried in the present authors' laboratory with elutes obtained from standardized cylinders of material (1.9 mm in diameter and 1 mm high) of Photac-Fil Aplicap, Vitremer, Fuji II LC, Dyract, and Compoglass. The eluates were tested on cultures of confluent pulp cells (second subculture) and on gingival and dermal cells (sixth and seventh subcultures). The following conclusions were reached.

- The most highly cytotoxic effect is obtained from eluates obtained within the first 3 days after extraction. The toxicity of the eluates decreased after 3 days for Vitremer and after 2 days for Hi-Dense, Fuji II LC, and Dyract. Eluate obtained with Compoglass was less cytotoxic than eluates obtained from other biomaterials.
- The concentration of the eluate plays a role in cytotoxicity. For example, Hi-Dense eluate is always cytotoxic, whatever the concentration. In contrast, Vitremer and Fuji II LC are cytotoxic at concentrations above 5%. Eluates from Photac-Fil, Dyract, and Compoglass are cytotoxic at concentrations above 5% and strongly cytotoxic at 10%.
- Only slight differences appear between the reactions observed in pulp cells and gingival cells. However, in some circumstances, pulp cells react very specifically.
- Preabsorption of the eluate on dentin powders firmly reduces the cytotoxicity of eluates.
- Because some cytotoxic components can be absorbed on dentin powder, potential agents were checked. The pHs of all the eluates were between 7.5 and 8, except for Hi-Dense and Vitremer, which were 5.9 and 6.3, respectively, for a 100% concentration. Hence, the pH was not related to the reaction.

- Fluoride and aluminum concentrations exerted a severe influence on pulp cells, but only above 1mm. Fluoride release by the biomaterials varied. At 100% concentration of the eluate, Compoglass did not release any fluoride. The same quantity was released by Photac-Fil, Vitremer, Fuji II LC, and Dyract, but Hi-Dense released twice as much.
- Zinc was toxic at concentration in the order of 0.01mm. Strontium was never cytotoxic at any concentration.
- These conclusions indicate that none of the parameters listed earlier are involved in cell cytotoxicity and therefore it is possible that some unpolymerized and leachable resin components are responsible for the cytotoxic reactions.

To compare the cytotoxicity of five RMGICs and one metal-reinforced GIC, Stanislawski, et al. carried out an *in vitro* pulp cell viability assay. The most toxic materials were the metal-reinforced GIC and RMGIC Vitremer (3M/ ESPE), while the least toxic were the RMGICs Compoglass (Ivoclar Vivadent Ltda., São Paulo, SP, Brasil) and Photac Fil (3M/ESPE). This toxicity was due to the presence ofunpolymerized monomers, such as HEMA and TEGDMA, and polyacrilic acid, which were leached from resin modified materials and metal-reinforced GIC. The main elements responsible for the toxicity of the metal-reinforced GIC were Cu2+ and Ag+ present in toxic concentrations. It was further analyzed the possible cytotoxicity of some ions that are present in significant amounts in GICs, such as F-, Al3+, Zn2+ and Sr2+. The zinc was the only component that was found to be of a sufficiently high concentration to induce cytotoxicity. These elements were present in the metalreinforced GIC and may have contributed to its cytotoxicity. Complementing the results presented above, the cytotoxic effects of five RMGICs and conventional GICs on an odontoblast cell line were studied. The GICs were the least cytotoxic experimental materials and the RMGICs caused intense cytophatic effects on the cultured cells decreasing significantly the cell metabolism as well as causing remarkable cell death. The high cytotoxic effects observed for RMGICs in that study may be caused by unreacted resin monomers rather than by other compounds such as F-, Al3+, Sr2+, Zn2+ which are present in the conventional GICs. Although a true RMGIC must be capable of setting without being light-activated45, higher levels of released HEMA are found when these cements are only allowed to cure chemically[4]. The liner RMGIC Vitrebond (3M/ESPE) releases a high concentration of HEMA monomer before immersion in distilled water, even when polymerized according to the manufacturer's recommendations, when compared to the amount released from the restorative RMGIC Vitremer (3M/ESPE)4. Other RMGIC toxic components, such as fluoride, aluminum, silver, siliceous, strontium, zinc and silicate, may also be released during the setting reaction or solubilization of the cement in a wet environment4, but it was already mentioned that the ions released from the RMGIC are not sufficiently high to cause cytotoxic effects, except for Zn2+ . Other studies affirm that conventional GICs are less cytotoxic than the RMGICs Vitrebond (3M/ESPE) and Vitremer (3M/ESPE), which caused intense cytophatic effects in cell cultures decreasing significantly the cell metabolism as well as causing remarkable cell death .The adverse effect caused by Vitremer (3M/ESPE) was attributed to the leaching of at least two components of polyacidic phase (HEMA) as well as unidentified acidic species. Other authors compared the toxicity of 9 types of GICs on cultured human dental pulp cells and concluded that RMGICs are more toxic to pulp cells than conventional GICs. Consequently, the application of RMGICs directly onto dental pulp cells is not recommended. However, current *in vivo* studies performed in human teeth have demonstrated that the RMGIC Vitrebond (3M/ESPE) applied as a liner in very deep class V cavities caused no inflammatory pulp response15,20. In this way, it seems that the presence of a dentin barrier between this kind of lightcured RMGIC and the pulp cells may prevent pulpal damage.[66]

Biocompatibility of glass-ionomer bone cements:

Due to their excellent biocompatibility in dental applications GIC have been formulated for medical applications. There is little doubt that GICs compare favourably with alternative bone cements for specific applications, based on in vitro and in vivo studies. The most important paper on the pathology responsible for the death of a patient following treatment with a glass-ionomer bone cement was provided by Reushe et al. in 2001.They reported that aluminium was detected in brain, CSF, urine and blood up to 77 d after surgery, although the aluminium content of brain tissue was less than commonly found in dialysis associated encephalopathy. They concluded that failure to close the dura was the primary reason for accumulation of aluminium in patient's brain. This was because 99 similar operations performed atWurzburg using a glass-ionomer bone cement showed no psychiatric or neurologic side effects.

Despite the evidence now suggesting good surgical technique can overcome the potential for toxicity of glass-ionomer bone cements in many applications, surgeons are understandably (and quite correctly) cautious.Concerns regarding the release of aluminium from glass-ionomershave ledto thedevelopment of aluminium-free compositions by workers at Sheffield. If these are shown to be biocompatible in vivo, in time they may form the basis of a new generation of medical grade glass ionomer bone cements.

Glasses with the following molar compositions were fabricated:

4.5SiO2_3M2O3_XP2O5_3CaO_2CaF2 (M = Al or Fe, X = 0–1.5). The glasses were characterised using X-ray fluorescence (XRF) and X-ray powder diffraction (XRD). Cements were prepared using a standard ratio of; 1 g of glass powder: 0.2 g of dried polyacrylic acid: 0.3 g of 10% tartaric acid solution. Cement formation was assessed using a Gilmore needle and in vitro biocompatibility was investigated for novel cement formulations. XRF revealed that the Fe2O3-based glasses had Al2O3 contamination from the crucibles and also had undergone substantial F_ losses. XRD gave peaks that corresponded to magnetite Fe3O4 (JCPDS # 19-629) in all compositions. Apatite Ca5(PO4)3(OH,F) (JCPDS # 15-876) was identified in P2O5 containing glasses. It was possible to fabricate cements from all of the Fe_2O_3-based ionomer glasses. Good in vitro biocompatibility was observed for the Fe_2O_3- based cements.[68]

Ionomer glasses may be prepared by entirely replacing Al_2O_3 with Fe_2O_3.
Cement setting times appeared to be related to P_2O_5 content. Fe_2O_3-based cements showed good in vitro biocompatibility.

Summary

Dental materials continue to evolve, and which material will finally prove optimal is unknown. It might be glass-ionomer cements or new materials formed from biological molecules that will heal wounded tissue at great speed or induce biological mineralization. At the moment, glass-ionomer cements are useful materials, especially those whose physical properties have been improved by the addition of resins. However, if these materials are going to replace others, it will first be necessary to have a better understanding of what happens in their interaction with pulp cells.

10. BONDING GLASS-IONOMER CEMENTS TO TOOTH STRUCTURE

Ten years ago it would have been relatively straightforward to write about the mechanisms of attachment of glass-ionomer cements to tooth tissue, but the same cannot be said today. In the intervening years, the field's understanding of the strengths and weaknesses of dental hard tissues has not changed greatly, but the range of materials related to the ionomeric setting reaction has greatly diversified. Briefly, the available glass-ionomer materials now range from highly water-sensitive acid-base cements to materials with setting reactions that are almost entirely resin based. Not surprisingly, the way they bond to tooth tissue may be profoundly affected by their resin content. To gain a full appreciation of their adhesive-substrate interactions it is first necessary to understand the relevant anatomy and physiology of the substrate itself.

The Substrate: Enamel and Dentin

To grossly simplify the situation, enamel is dry and brittle, dentin is wet and resilient. Enamel is an immensely strong bio-material but does have inherent planes of weakness, a fact not often appreciated in the literature for adhesive dental materials. The basic structural unit of enamel is the hydroxyapatite crystal. Approximately 10,000 of these long, slender crystals are packed closely together to form a 7 µm diameter prism or rod. This unit extends from the enamel-dentin junction (EDJ) to the surface of the tooth, a distance of up to 2.5 mm. The hydroxyapatite crystals can be very long in comparison to their width, behaving rather like the fibers in a rope; this, in conjunction with the complexity of the prism shape and course, leads to an extremely tough and hard-wearing material. Such strength is, however, highly directional in this anisotropic material. The prism unit is very difficult to pull and break on its long axis because of the crystal orientation. The optimal enamel prism orientation for bonding is therefore on the long axis. Attachment to the sides of prisms is less satisfactory. Prisms can, however, bent laterally and ruptured by weaker forces than are required for breakage on the long axis. Such prism orientations are readily encountered in the lateral walls of proximal cavities.

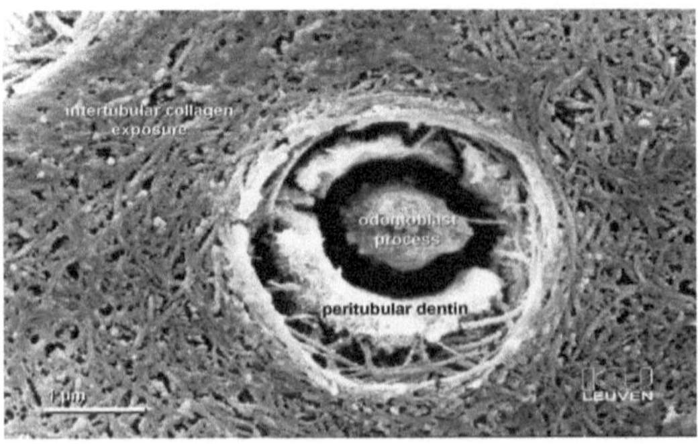

The above Fe-SEM photomicrograph illustrates the effect of a polyalkenoic acid conditioner (Cavity Conditioner, GC) that was applied for 10 s on dentin covered by a smear layer. Although intertubular dentin was exposed, hydroxyapatite was not completely removed from collagen and remained as receptors for additional chemical interaction. Micro-pores were created to enable micro-mechanical interlocking through hybridisation.

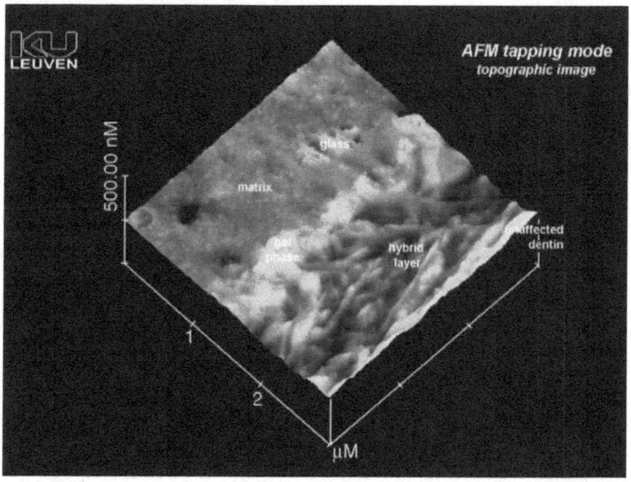

Atomic force microscopy photomicrograph illustrating the 3D-topography of the interface between the resin-modified glass-ionomer Fuji Bond LC and dentin (tapping mode)

A major structural unit of dentin is the dentin tubule, running from the EDJ to the pulp. This 1- to 2-µm-diameter tubule, conveys pulpal fluid from the pulp to the enamel, maintaining the hydration of the tooth and other physiologic functions. The inherent outward flow of fluid profoundly reduces the penetration of adhesives into the tubules and may have an effect on water-sensitive cements. Tubule density at the EDJ is 19,000mm^2 and increases toward the pulp to 45,000mm^2. The diameter of the tubule also increases from 0.8 µm at the EDJ to 2.5µm at the pulp. It is therefore self-evident that deeper dentin is much "wetter" than that at the periphery of the tooth, affecting the performance of water sensitive restorative materials.

In the outer two thirds of the dentin, the tubule itself is surrounded by a thin coating of highly mineralized peritubular dentin. The bulk of this coating consists of a matrix of type 1 collagen embedded in hydroxyapatite crystals to form the intertubular dentin. Hypermineralization of dentin occurs a normal response to caries and tooth wear and, by reducing permeability, confers a protective function by preventing noxious substances from entering the pulp.

Dentin is neither strong nor weak in any particular direction; compared to enamel it is isotropic. It can therefore be appreciated that dentin is a multiphase material which presents many problems for bonding due to its water content, its resilience and its inhomogeneity.

Enamel and dentin are intimately related to each other with a scalloped interface at the EDJ. The enamel protects dentin from wear, and the dentin supports the brittle enamel. Without adequate support from the dentin, the enamel shell is easily lost: examples of this are situations in which the dentin structure is defective, as in dentinogenesis imperfecta or in dentinal caries. Many of the crack-stopping features within enamel, such as prism decussation and the sinuous nature of the prisms in the inner two thirds of the enamel, commence at the EDJ.

Cutting these hard tissues produces a structure called the *smear layer(* < 20μm thick) on both the enamel and dentin. This is more or less well attached to the tooth surface and consists of cutting debris, which is pressure-welded to the tooth. It has the effect of reducing fluid outflow from the dentin by plugging the tubular openings. Due to its brittleness, cutting enamel introduces subsurface cracks and fault lines, which can lead to structural weakness if adhesive materials are bonded to this damaged substrate.

Nondestructive microscopic imaging

Scanning optical, or confocal, microscopy offers many advantages for imaging tooth tissue and glass-ionomer cements, because of the ability of the investigator to control their water content and also to examine undisturbed structures below the section surface. Further information can be gained by consulting specific references.

General Requirements for Adhesion

The general perceived requirements for adhesion are expounded in many dental textbooks. Good substrate wetting, a low contact angle, and a clean substrate are normally considered essential. The surface tension of the liquid adhesive must always be less than the surface energy of the enamel or dentin. The contamination of the tooth surface by saliva, blood, or other proteinaceous substances reduces the surface energy of the substrate and impairs wetting by the liquid adhesive. Put simply, the first thing to touch a "clean" tooth surface, whether saliva or bonding resin, makes the strongest bond.

The most likely mechanisms of bonding to tooth structure are as follows:

- Mechanical theories that involve the concept of interlocking the solidified adhesive with the irregularities of the adherent surface.
- Adsorption theories that comprise all the explanations involving chemical bonding and similar forces between the adhesive and adherent. The forces involved may be primary (ionic

and covalent) and secondary (hydrogen, dipole interaction, or Van der Waals') valence forces.

- Diffusion theories that involve the concept of bonding between mobile molecules across the interface.

Following these criteria, it would be easy to appreciate that the enamel-composite bond falls into the first category: the tooth surface is etched and dried, and free-flowing fluid resin is placed and cured. A viscous glass-ionomer cement may fall into the second and third categories because, even without acid etching of the tooth, conventional glass-ionomer cements are inherently adhesive restorations compared with the resin composites. It would appear that there must be other mechanisms at work.

Adhesion can be achieved in a number of different ways and much of the literature has speculated on the attachment of conventional glass-ionomers to teeth. Much of this is based on concepts of polar dispersion, ionic diffusion, and alterations to surface topography and surface energies.

Adhesion Mechanisms of Conventional Glass-Ionomer Cements

The development of the tooth - glass ionomer bond evolves over time. Unlike resin-based systems, the bond strength increases to become eventually limited by the cohesive tensile strength of the cement rather than by its adhesive strength alone.

The initial attraction between the cut tooth and freshly placed cement is mainly due to polar attraction, with weak hydrogen bonds predominating. At this stage, the acidity of the cement, allows it to act as a self-etching agent on the tooth smear layer. The hydrogen ions are rapidly buffered by the phosphate ions from the hydroxyapatite crystals, but widespread exposure of collagen is limited because of the weakness of the acids involved. Even if the cement is relatively viscous, the watery environment of the tooth and the free water in the cement should ensure an ionic exchange at the interface. In this way, good wetting of the substrate by the adhesive is achieved. Water flux at the dentin interface is indicated by the transfer of dye from the cement as a fluorescent band, as imaged using confocal microscopy.

The continuing development of the bond is thought to be caused by further movement of ionic species in the interface, perhaps due to diffusion as the phosphate ions are displaced by the polyalkenoic acids. This theory suggests that to maintain an electrolytic balance it is necessary for each phosphate ion to take with it a calcium ion. These are then taken up by the cement adjacent to the tooth to produce an ion- enriched layer that is firmly bound to both enamel and dentin. The strength of both the ion-enriched layer and its union to the tooth have yet to be measured.

Maximum achievable bond strength for glass-ionomers is only reached after the cement has undergone its maturation process. On addition of the liquid to the powder, hardening occurs due to attack of the glass surface by hydronium ions (hydrated protons of the acid), causing the release of calcium and aluminum ions. The ions form salt bridges between carboxyl groups of the polyacid; resulting in a gel matrix surrounding the intact glass particles. The maturation of glass-ionomer restorations is relatively slow. In the initial stages of the setting reaction, divalent calcium ions are released rapidly and form primarily calcium salt bridges between polyacrylate chains within the cement. Such salt bridges also form at the interface with hydroxyapatite in the tooth. At this stage, both water uptake and water loss can occur, with the attendant clinical problems of contamination and dehydration. Provisions must be made to maintain the water balance of restorations for the first 24 hours. In later stages of the setting reaction, cross-linking by trivalent aluminum ions gives greater stability to the matrix structure.

At full maturation, the cement at the interface will have become very viscous and its initial reactions with the tooth substrate will have ensured a close adaptation. Minimal setting movements of the cement, if it is kept fully hydrated, will also maintain the close approximation of tooth and cement to allow further ion exchange to occur over the lifetime of the restoration.

Glass – ionomer cements, as many research workers have shown have the important property of permanently adhering to untreated enamel and dentine under the moist conditions of the mouth. They share this property with the zinc polycarboxylate cements. Whether the cement penetrates the acquired pellicle on enamel or bonds to it is uncertain, but it does react with the smear layer on cut dentine. This is an important attribute for a filling material and, to a lesser degree, for a luting agent. Glass-ionomer cements also bond to other reactive polar substrates, such as the base metals.

Acid etching or other surface-roughening procedures are deprecated, for the bonding is of a chemical rather than a micromechanical nature. About 80% of maximum bond strength is developed in 15 minutes (Aboush and Jenkins, 1986), but strength slowly increases for several days after that (Powis et al., 1982).

Tensile bond strengths (MPa) of glass-ionomer cements to untreated enamel and dentine

Material	Enamel	Dentine
ASPA IV	2.6, 3.2	1.5, 3.1
De Trey Aspa	3.6, 4.8, 4.5	1.8, 2.4 1.1 4.0
	4.5, 5.2	2.4, 2.4, 3.3[m]
Chem. – Filt	9.6	4.1[m]
Chembond	4.8	1.3[d], 2.3[e]
Fuji lonomer	4.5, 4.5, 4.2	2.5[e], 4.5[k], 2.2[i], 3.1[m]
Ketac – Cem	4.2	2.2[f]
Detac – Fai	6.4	3.3[m]

Shear bond strengths (MPa) of glass – ionomer cements to untreated enamel and dentine

Material	Enamel	Dentine
De Trey Aspa*	1.6[a]	6.8[c], 4.0[d], 4.0[e]
Fuji ionomer ‖+	4.2[b]	2.4[f], 3.3[b]

Adhesion is the most important property of the glass-inomer cement. It allows a conservative approach to restoration, because undercutting to provide mechanical keying is unnecessary in low–stress-bearing areas. This is of particular advantage in restoring cervical erosion lesions and in sealing pits and fissures (McLean and Wilson, 1974, 1977, 1977b).

Adhesion to dentine and enamel enables the glass-inomer cement to provide a perfect seal. Bearing in mind that the percolation of bacteria along the cavity wall/restoration interface has been cited as the cause of pulpal inflammation (Brannstorm, 1981) it follows that adhesion has important implications for biocompatibility.

Barriers to adhesion :

The principal barrier to effective adhesion to dental tissue is water. Dentine is permeated by aqueous fluids transported from the pulp, and there is both loosely and tightly bound water in the surface of enamel. In the oral situation, organic adhesives are either insufficiently polar to compete with water for the surface of dental tissue, or, if highly polar, the bond they form is hydrolytically unstable. By contrast, the hydrophilic, highly ionic glass-ionmer cement competes successfully with water because of its multiplicity of carboxyl groups that form hydrogen bonds with the substrate. Water is displaced or even incorporated into the cement. Adhesion is permanent, because of the multiplicity of hydrogen and ionic bonds that attach the glas-ionomer cement to the substrate in an octopuslike fashion, making temporary scission of one such bond inconsequential.

Another barrier to adhesion is the dynamic nature of tooth material. Because enamel is an ion exchanger and dentine is a living material subject to change, one is trying to bond to shifting sand rather than to solid rock. Under such conditions the adhesive bond must have a dynamic character too. It will be broken as the substrate changes, and must be capable of being re-formed. Once broken, covalent chemical bonds cannot be re-formed. Dentine adhesives may fail because of this very point. By contrast, the ionic and polar bonds that attach the glass-ionomer cement to the substrate can be re-established, which, together with the multiplicity of the adhesive bonds, may account for this cement's unique property of being permanently adhesive under oral conditions. [4]

Mechanism of adhesion to enamel and dentine :

The precise mechanism of adhesion of polyelectrolyte cements has yet to be fully elucidated. Several hypotheses have been advanced. It is certain that the adhesive bond is a chemical one affected by chemical and not mechanical factors.

Chemically, tooth material consists of apatite, which makes up over 98% of enamel and 70% of dentine by weight, and collagen which is found in dentine alone (McLean, 1980). The bond of glass-ionomer cement to enamel is better than to dentine – evidence that bonding to apatite is the principal mode of adhesion. If the cement bonds mainly to the apatite constituent of dentine with little or no bonding to collagen then the bond strength will be lowered but there will be no adhesive failure at the apatite sites. This may explain the general observation that the failure of bonds to dentine, like those to enamel, is adhesive rather than cohesive.

Smith (1968) speculated that chelation of calcium, contained in apatite, was involved in adhesion, but Beech (1973) considered this mechanism was unlikely as it would involve the formation of an eight-membered ring. Instead he proposed, on the basis of an infrared spectroscopic study, that the interaction between apatite and poly(acrylic acid) produced polyacrylate ions which then formed strong ionic bonds with the surface calcium ions of apatite in enamel and dentine.

Wilson (1974) looked at the mechanism of adhesion more broadly. He suggested that initially, when the cement paste is applied to tooth material and is fluid, wetting and initial adhesion is by hydrogen bonding provided by free carboxyl groups present in the fresh paste.As the cement ages, hydrogen bonds are progressively replaced by ionic bonds, the cations coming either from the cement or the hydroxyapatite. Wilson stressed the important role of the polyelectrolyte moiety, for the older phosphate-bonded cements, unlike the polyelectrolyte cements, do not adhere to tooth substances. It follows that the polymeric polar chains of polyacid are essential for the achievement of adhesion. Their role must be one of bridging the interface between the cement and the substrate, a role that isolated orthophosphate ions cannot assume.

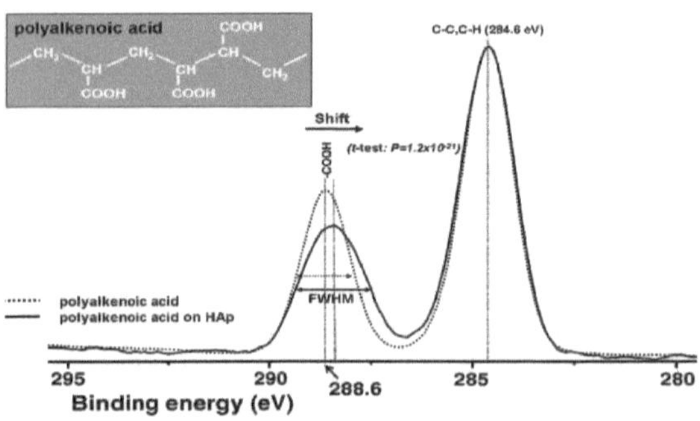

XPS narrow-scan spectra of the C 1s region of the acrylic/maleic polyalkenoic acid co-polymer and of the polyalkenoic acid applied on hydroxyapatite. Interaction of the polyalkenoic acid with hydroxyapatite resulted in a significant shift of the peak representing the carboxyl groups (–COO*S*) to a lower binding energy, suggesting the formation of an ionic bond to hydroxyapatite.

More recently, Wilson, Prosser, and Powis (1983), on the basis of adsorption and infrared spectroscopic studies, postulated that, during adsorption, polyacrylate entered the molecular surface of hydroxyapatite, displacing and replacing surface phosphate. Calcium ions are displaced from hydroxyapatite along with phosphate as part of a complex series of ionic exchanges. These workers inferred that, as a consequence of these interactions, an intermediate layer of calcium and aluminim phosphates and polyacrylates would form at the interface between the cement and apatite. Interestingly, much earlier, McLean and Wilson (1977 a) had partly anticipated this model when they hypothesized on the presence of an intermediate interfacing layer between cement and tooth surface.

Chain length must also be an important factor in adhesion. The dental silicate cement does not bond to tooth tissue, although nearly all arguments applied to glass-ionomer adhesion apply to the silicate also. The difference is that whereas the dental silicate cement is an assembly of discrete cations and phosphate anions, the glass-ionomer cement is based on a polymer chain that is capable of bridging gaps between the cement body and the substrate.

While there is general agreement that bonding to enamel, which is almost entirely apatite, results from ionic and polar forces, there is no consensus of opinion on bonding to dentine, which contains a large proportion of the organic constituent collagen. Beech (1973) maintained that bonding only, citing the weaker adhesion of the glass-ionomer cement to dentine and the nonexistence of adhesion to decalcified dentine. Wilson (1974) considered the possibility of polyacrylates bonding to collagen also. Collagen contains both amino and carboxylic acid groups, so there could be adhesion by hydrogen bonding or cationic bridges. Recent adsorption studies at the Laboratory of the Government Chemist, however, indicate that poly(acrylic acid) and polyacrylate are not absorbed on collagen (Jackson, 1986). The probability is that glass-ionomer cements do not bond to collagen.

Evidence is accumulating that bond strength to tooth substances depends on the nature of the polyacid used. Cements based on poly(acrylic acid) appear to bond more strongly than those based on copolymers of acrylic acid with itaconic or maleic acids (Aboush and Jenkins, 1986). If this proves to be so then the molecular configuration of the polyacid would be an important factor in controlling adhesion.

Only one study on the adhesion of cermet cements has been reported (Thronton et al., 1986). Research workers found that the adhesion of a cermet cement to enamel and dentine was inferior to that of a conventional glass-inomer cement, a result that was attributed to poorer flow properties. They suggested that mechanical keying may be necessary. Powis (1986) recommended the pretreatment of enamel and dentine with poly (acrylic acid), which is not subsequently washed off, so that a bonding intermediary is formed.

Improving adhesion :

When the cement tooth bond fractures it is by cohesive failure within the cement rather than adhesive failure at the interface. Thus, the strength of the bond is limited by the cohesive strength of the cement used.

The tensile bond strength to enamel is greater than that to dentine ; the bond strength to enamel varies from 2.6 to 9.6 MPa, depending on the material, and from 1.1 to 4.5 MPa to cut but untreated dentine. Interestingly, bonding is achieved to both enamel and dentine without any sort of surface treatment, although a smear layer is present on the surface of cut enamel and dentine. Indeed, this layer may be beneficial if it is consolidated. However, Prodger and Symonds (1977) reported that salivary contamination of a freshly prepared dentine surface reduce bond strength, but whether this was because of its water content or contamination of the dentine surface is uncertain.[14]

Surface conditioning:

A number of research workers have sought to improve adhesion. One way that is common to nearly all adhesive technologies is by pretreatment of the surface. McLean and Wilson (1977b) first used the term surface conditioning for this treatment in order to differentiate it from acid etching. Surface conditioning is needed in order to eliminate the wide variation found in the structures of tooth surfaces following cutting. The case for surface treatment, however, is still one of controversy. The issue is unlikely to be finally resolved until stronger glass-ionomer cements are available to make distinctions clearer. However, on one point all agree : rough tooth surfaces are contraindicated. In general, the smoother the surface the stronger the bond, and this is not a marginal effect (Powis et al., 1982 ; Aboush and Jenkins, 1986). Indeed, the smoothing of the cut dentine and enamel surfaces may be the mechanism whereby surface conditioners improve adhesion, for the most effective surface conditioners, as will be shown, while having different actions on tooth surfaces, all tend to smooth it. Good interfacial contact is important for adhesion. The smoothing of surface irregularities may be necessary to prevent air entrapment and to minimize sites where stress concentration could occur.

The majority of investigators find that surface conditioners improve bond strength, especially to dentine; a few maintain that there is no effect (Prodger and Symonds, 1977; Beech et al., 1985). Rarely is reduction in bond strength reported. In the nature of things one would expect both positive and negative effects from surface treatments. If the whole body of evidence is accepted, then the very fact that there are differences between research workers, who use a variety of techniques and operate on teeth of varying natures, indicates that the condition of the surface is important. It would appear logical that if a surface treatment is proven never to be deleterious then it should be used in all cases for the condition of teeth and the techniques of operators will vary widely. The perfect surface treatment would be one that eliminated all these variables.

Again, these surface treatments are conditioning treatments and are to be distinguished from the etching techniques used for bonding composite resins to enamel. Surface demineralization, associated with etching techniques, is undesirable and deprecated for the bonding of glass-ionomer cements to dentine and enamel (Powis et al., 1982). Decalcifying freshly cut dentine opens up and widens dentinal tubules, allowing ingress of bacteria, and so causing inflammation (Brannstorm, 1981)[4].

Effect of various surface conditioners on the bond strengths (MPa) of ASPA IV to enamel and dentine

Surface treatment	Time of application (seconds)	Enamel	Dentine
None	-	3.2	3.1
Citric acid, 50% aq	30	5.6	3.7
Citric acid, 2% aq/alc	30	5.6	3.7
Poly (acrylic acid), 25% aq	30	7.1	6.8
Tannic acid, 25% aq	60	7.0	6.3
Surface – active solution ‡	60	7.5	6.6
Dodicin, 0.9% aq	60	6.3	6.3
Na_2 EDTA, 2% aq	30	5.0	2.1
Na_4 EDTA, 15% aq	30	5.3	1.9
Sodium fluoride, 3% aq	30	4.7	4.8
Ferric chloride, 2% aq/alc	30	4.5	5.4

Effect of various surface conditioners on the bond strengths (MPa) of glass-ionomer cements to dentine

Surface conditioner	Cement	Conditioned	No treatment	Investigators*
Poly (acrylic acid)	ASPA IV ‡	6.8	3.1	Powis et al. (1982)t
Poly (acrylic acid)	Fuji ionomer II‡	2.7	2.2	Beech et al. (1985)t
Ferric chloride	ASPA IV	5.4	3.1	Powis et al. (1982)t
Ferric chloride	De Trey Aspa §	4.7	2.2	Shalabi et al. (1981)t
ITS	De Trey Aspa	6.0	4.0	Causton & Johnson (1982)s
ITS	Fuji ionomer II	3.3	2.2	Beech et al. (1985)t
Mineralizing solution	De Trey Aspa	4.8	2.4	Levine et al. (1979)t

Citric acid :

The earliest surface conditioner for the bonding of glass-ionomer cements to tooth substrates, proposed by McLean and Wilson (1977a, 1977b), was citric acid (50%), which was chosen because of its compatibility with the cement – citric acid is a cement-former. It has had its advocates (Hotz et al., 1977; vliestra et al., 1978; Prodger and Symonds, 1977) and its detractors (Cotton and Siegal, Vougiouklakis et al., 1982; Hood et al., 1977). Its use has fallen into some disfavour but it is still commonly employed in adhesive studies for comparative purposes. It generally increases bond strength or has no effect. On these grounds its use cannot be deprecated, although there are now better surface conditioners available.

There has also been controversy over the effectiveness of citric acid on the bonding of the glass-ionomer cement to dentine. However, this controversy has now been resolved and again illustrates the danger of generalizing on the basis of limited experiments. The nature of the bonding to dentine is now known to depend on the particular glass-inomer cement used (Vougiouklakis et al., 1982). Glass-ionomer cements adhere to citric acid-treated dentine by two mechanisms : chemical bonding and micromechanical attachment to the opened-up-tubules. In the case of De Trey Aspa (based on a copolymer of itaconic and acrylic acid) the gain of bonding by micromechanical attachment exceeded the loss brought about by partial decalcification of dentine. The reverse was found to be true for poly (acrylic acid) – based Fuji inomer II. Thus, the appropriateness of the surface treatment depends on the material used.

Although not a strong acid, citric acid can be extremely erosive because of its ability to chelate metal ions. Powis et al. (1982) found that the effect of citric acid was drastic, with the surfaces of both dentine and enamel being attacked. The enamel surface was heavily etched, as comparison of show. The smear layer was removed from dentine and the dentinal tubules were opened up with loss of perihedral dentine. Optimum adhesion was not achieved with this severe treatment. Removal of the smear layer and the opening of tubules can lead to demineralization and hence decrease the chemical interaction of the cement with the tooth. For this reason Brannstrom (1981) advocates a treatment time of only five seconds.

Other surface conditioners :

The most extensive study of surface conditioners was made by Powis et al. (1982), who examined a range of surface treatments, including simple cleansers and chelating polyfunctional carboxylic and phenolic acids, using adhesion tests and scanning electron microscopy.

Bond strengths (MPa) of glass-ionomer cements to untreated and citric acid-conditioned enamel*

Investigators	Cement	No treatment	Citric acid
Hotz et al. (1977)	ASPA IV‡	2.9	4.1
Powis et al. (1982)	ASPA IV	3.2	5.6
Prodger & Symonds (1977)	De Trey Aspa ‡	3.6	3.2
Lacefield et al. (1982)	Fuji ionomer ‖§	4.5	5.0
Aboush & Jenkins (1986)	De Trey Aspa	5.2	5.9
Aboush & Jenkins (1986)	Chem.-Fil ¶	9.6	9.9
Aboush & Jenkins (1986)	Ketac – Fil #	6.4	6.1
Aboush & Jenkins (1986)	Fuji ionomer II	4.2	4.8

Bond strengths (MPa) of glass-ionomer cements to untreated and citric-acid-conditioned dentine

Investigators*	Cement	No treatment	Citric acid
Hotz et al. (1977)t	ASPA IV‡	1.5	2.9
Powis et al. (1982)t	ASPA Iv	3.1	3.7
Prodger & Symonds (1977)t	De Trey Aspa ‡	1.8	1.7
Hood et al., (1977)s	De Trey Aspa	6.8	4.1
Shalabi et al. (1983)t	De Trey Aspa	2.2	1.9
Negm et al., (1982)t	De Trey Aspa	2.4	1.6
Lacefield et al. (1982)t	Fuji ionomer II§	3.3	2.5
Aboush & Jenkins (1986)t	De Trey Aspa	1.8	3.3
Aboush & Jenkins (1986)t	Chem.-Fil ¶	2.3	4.1
Aboush & Jenkins (1986)t	Ketac-Fil#	1.6	3.3

Powis et al. (1982) found other treatments to be more effective than citric acid. The best agents for improving adhesion to enamel and dentine proved to be 25% poly (acrylic acid), 25% tannic acid, and a surface-active detergent, 0.9% dodicin, which contains fluoride. These treatments had different effects on the surfaces of dentine and enamel, but all were equally as effective as and less disruptive than citric acid.

Mount (1984) has suggested that surface conditioners should, ideally, meet the following requirements :

1. Be isotonic to minimize osmotic effects
2. Have a pH ranging from 5.5 to 8.0 that is, be broadly neutral
3. Be nontoxic to dentine, pulp, and gingival tissues
4. Be compatible with the chemistry of the cement
5. Have water solubility and be easily removed
6. Not deplete enamel and dentine chemically
7. Enhance the surface chemically in preparation for bonding

Of course, not all of these criteria can be met, and it is not certain whether they always need to be fully met. This useful advice may be extended and amended. Acidic solutions are not the only chemical substances to decalcify enamel and dentine-neutral complexing agents can have a similar effect. However, when these acid and complexing agents form insoluble cementitious substances, their adverse effect is negated. The increase in bonding efficiency must be attributed in part to (1) a 'cleaning' effect, by which loose cutting debris is removed, to (2) a partial 'demineralization' effect, bywhichthe surface area is increased and micro-porosities for micro-mechanical interlocking or hybridisation are exposed, but also in part to (3) chemical interaction of the polyalkenoic acid with residual hydroxyapatite (see further).Anetwork of 'hydroxyapatite-coated' collagen fibrils interspersed by pores is typically exposed up to a depth of no deeper than 1 mm. Transmission electron microscopy (TEM) and X-ray photo-electron spectroscopy (XPS) have demonstrated that (though depending on the product) this polyalkenoic acid is usually not completely rinsed off. An upto 0.5 mm thick layer, often referred to as 'gel phase', remains attached to the tooth surface despite the conditioner is being rinsed off . The auto-adhesion of glass-ionomers to tooth tissue has recently been elucidated to be two-fold in nature. Micromechanical interlocking is achieved by shallow hybridisation.

of the micro-porous, hydroxyapatite-coated collagen fibril network . In this respect, glass-ionomers can be considered as adhering to tooth tissue through a kind of selfetch approach. The basic difference with the resin-based selfetch approach is that glass-ionomers are self-etching through the use of a relatively high molecular weight (8000–20 000) polycarboxyl-based polymer. Resin-based self-etch adhesives make use of acidic low-MW monomers.

As the second part of the self-adhesion mechanism, true primary chemical bonding occurs through the formation of ionic bonds between the carboxyl groups of the polyalkenoic acid and calcium of hydroxyapatite that remained around the exposed surface collagen . This was proven for polyalkenoic acids applied to hydroxyapatite, but also to enamel as well as dentin.5 It was also demonstrated that the actual molecular formula of the polyalkenoic acid significantly influences the chemical bonding potential. XPS clearly showed that a polyalkenoic acid based upon 10:1 acrylic/maleic acid units has about two third of its carboxyl groups bonded to hydroxyapatite versus only half of the carboxyl groups of pure polyacrylic acid. Typical of some glass-ionomers is the morphologic manifestation of the 'gel-phase' at the interface, as it was shown correlatively by transmission electron microscopy and atomic force microscopy . Correlating TEM and XPS data has elucidated that this gel phase represents the formation of a calcium polycarboxylate salt resulting from either the polyalkenoic acid conditioner or the glassionomer material itself. This phase has been shown to be a stable and strong phase, intermediary between the shallow 0.5–1 mm hybrid layer and the glass-ionomer matrix. In micro-tensile bond strength testing, the interface typically fractures well above the gel phase within the matrix of the glass-ionomer material. The actual function and contribution of this phase to the bond integrity needs to be further elucidated.

Surface – active microbicidal solutions :

Powis et al. (1982) examined the use of the old – style Tubulicid* formulations (0.1% chlorhexidine gluconate; 0.08% dodicin; 3% sodium fluoride), both with and without ^{fluoride}, as surface conditioners. These are approximately neutral solutions and a 60-second treatment produces no adverse effects. Results are given in Table 6-3. The fluoride containing version produces the best results on both enamel and dentine. This surface conditioner appears to be as effective an adhesion promoter as poly (acrylic acid) and tannic acid.

The active conditioning agents appear to be dodicin, a surface-active agent, and fluoride. (It should be emphasized that currently available Tubulicid is of a different composition and its effectiveness is unknown.) When applied to enamel it smoothes out the ragged edges of grooves and removes debris produced by polishing. On dentine it smoothes out polishing grooves and, although dentinal tubules can be seen beneath a reduced smear layer, the tubules are not opened up. The solution is not chemically compatible with the cement system but is readily washed off.

Dodicin :

The surface – active agent dodicin by itself produces effects on dentine and enamel similar to the surface-active microbicidal solutions (Powis et al., 1982). Remarks in the previous section apply here.

Poly (acrylic acid) :

Poly (acrylic acid) in 25% aqueous solution was recommended as an effective surface conditioner by Powis et al. (1982). Because poly (acrylic acid) complexes metal ions and is also acidic, its solutions have a decalcifying action. For this reason, Mount (1984) recommends a short application time of 10 seconds. Its action is less drastic than that of citric acid, but it does etch enamel slightly while removing polishing marks. On cut dentine, its general effect is to remove surface debris and smooth out surface irregularities, although it does open up dentinal tubules.

We are tempted to say that poly (acrylic acid) is the conditioner of choice because it is part of the cement-forming system. Indeed, it must be used for the bonding of cermet cements, because the formation of an intermediate bonding layer between the restoration and the cavity wall is essential. However, there must be some reservation about its use on dentine, since, like citric acid, it opens the tubules. There is the possibility that this could lead to sensitivity, especially with luting agents. Although poly (acrylic acid) will not penetrate tubules because of its high molecular weight, opened tubules may offer a route for the movement of water.

Long et al. (1986) found that the optimum concentraction for poly (acrylic acid) lies between 30% to 35% and cited results which show a bond strength of 3.9 MPa with 35% poly (acrylic acid) against 3.0 MPa obtained with a 25% concentration.

Tannic acid:

Tannic acid, as its name implies, is an organic tanning agent. It reacts with collagen. Since it is also known to form cements with aluminosilicate glasses (Wilson, 1968), it would appear to have potential to couple the cement to collagen and so have advantages as a surface conditioner, at least for dentine, Powis et al. (1982) have found that tannic acid in 25% aqueous solution is at least as effective a surface conditioner as poly (acrylic acid) Tannic acid has an acidic reaction (pH = 2.5) and is not isotonic. Powis et al.(1982) recommend a 30- second period for treatment. When applied to enamel it forms a smooth featureless surface with out etching or decalcification. On dentine it also forms a smooth featureless layer and tubules are not opened but appear as blisters. Tannic acid probably undergoes a tanning reaction with collagen and so serves to consolidate the smear layer (Vaidyanthan et al., (1984).

Tannic acid could well be considered the material of choice for treating dentine because it forms a protective layer and dose not open up tubules. It could prove to be the answer to the problem of sensitivity sometimes found when the glass-ionomer cement is used as a luting agent, but this has yet to be proved. In effect it would be acting as a lining agent.

Ferric chloride :

The use of ferric chloride as a surface conditioner has been investigated by Powis et al. (1982), who used a 2% aqueous/alcoholic solution, and Shalai et al. (1981). Ferric chloride is an inorganic tanning agent and a mordant and is probably capable of being incorporated into both apatite and glass-ionomer cement. It has potential to provide metal linkages between collagen and glass-ionomer cement. It is also very acidic; ferric chloride hydrolyzes to give free hydrochloric acid, an acid stronger than phosphoric acid. Thus, its effect on enamel is dramatic, producing a surface with extensive fissuring, although whether this surface is the enamel or a reaction product is uncertain.

When ferric chloride is applied to dentine a unique surface is formed. Polishing grooves are almost obliterated but dentinal tubules are not exposed. Fissures are apparent in the surface but these are probably in a deposited coating rather than in the dentine itself. Although bond strengths are high, its use cannot be recommended in light of our present knowledge and its highly acidic nature. There could be a future in the treatment if an iron-containing complex is prepared that has a tanning action without the acidity of ferric chloride.

Sodium fluoride :

Somewhat surprisingly, Powis and coworkers (1982) found that sodium fluoride strengthened the adhesive bond both to enamel and dentine. Hydrogen bonds to fluoride are known to be the strongest hydrogen bonds and so this result, namely that fluoride enhances adhesion, supports the view that hydrogen bonding is of importance in adhesion.

Mineralizing solutions :

Mineralizing solutions have been developed by both Causton and Johnson (1979, 1982) – the ITS solution – and Levine et al. (1977), although Beech and coworkers (1985) consider these treatments ineffective. These solutions are approximately neutral and are isotonic. Details of preparation are given below.

This solution is prepared by mixing two stable solutions, A and B. Solution A is a 0.5 mol/l solution of potassium dihydrogen phosphate (pH = 4.5) saturated with brushite (calcium hydrogen phosphate dihydrate). Solution B is a 0.5 mol/l solution of disodium hydrogen phosphate (pH = 9) containing 2,000 ppm fluoride.

ITS solution:

Composition of the ITS solution is in g/L; application time is two minutes and shelf life is 18 months (refrigerated).

$CaCl_2 = 0.2$
$KCI = 0.2$
$MgCl_2.6H_2O = 0.5$
$NaCl = 8.0$
$NaHCO_3 = 1.0$
$NaH_2PO_2.H_2O = 0.05$
Glucose = 1.0

The object of these treatments is to promote mineralization of the dentine and increase the concentrations of calcium and phosphate ions within the smear layer. The time of application is two to three minutes, a relatively long one.

These workers found mineralizing treatments more effective for the zinc polycarboxylate cements than for the glass-inonomer cements. The relative ineffectiveness of these treatments on glass-ionomer cement is probably releated to calcium and phosphate in the cement and the formation of a calcium and phophate-rich layer between the cement and the tooth surface (Wilson et al., 1983). Obviously, further work is needed on these systems, but the same result might be achieved with modifications in the cement formulation.

EDTA :

Ethylenediaminetetracetic acid (EDTA) is an extremely powerful complexing agent for metal ions-more so than citric acid. It is a weak acid, almost insoluble in water, and so is used in the form of soluble sodium salts; the Na_2EDTA half-salt is approximately neutral, and the Na_4EDTA salt is alkaline in solution. Both are strong decalcifying agents because of the strong, soluble chelates they form with calcium . The effect of solutions of EDTA on dentine and enamel surfaces is broadly similar to that of citric acid. This decalcifying effect is reflected in the observation that they reduce the bond strength of glass-ionomer cement to dentine. Their use on dentine and enamel is, therefore, deprecated. Moreover, solutions of Na_4EDTA will attack the matrix of the glass-ionomer cement itself and so are incompatible with it. Therefore, their use as surface conditioners is to be deprecated.

Marginal leakage :

In recent years following the increasing interest in biocompatibility, attention has been focused on attaining an efficient marginal seal. A gap at the margin between a restoration and the cavity wall can result in the percolation of harmful microorganisms and chemicals that can give rise to secondary caries beneath the restoration. Adhesion of glass-ionomer cement to enamel and dentine led to the expectation that this cement would act as an efficient seal.

The expectation has been borne out by a number of workers using different in vitro methods of assessment (hembree and Andrews, 1978, Kidd, 1978; Maldonado et al., 1978; Powis et al., 1985; Gordon et al., 1986). Powis et al., (1985) found that glass-ionomer cements effected a permanent seal against the diffusion of sucrose (radiolabeled) for at least a year. No other restorative material was as effective, and all, including the etched composite resins, allowed leakage to some extent.

In addition, carious lesions in adjacent enamel have been shown to be reduced ; Kidd (1978) attributed this result to fluoride released by the cement being taken up by the enamel.

Good interfacial contact is important for adhesion. The smoothing of surface irregularities may be necessary to prevent air entrapment and to minimize sites where stress concentration could occur. Clearly, the most effective conditioners are those capable of forming hydrogen bonds with the tooth surface, so aiding wetting. They may also serve to consolidate the smear layer. Currently we recommend a ten-second application of a 25% solution of poly (acrylic acid) for the surface conditioning of cavities of dentine are involved, as in crown preparation.

The idea that surface smoothness is important comes from the recent work of Aboush and Jenkins (1986), who showed that bond strength decreased as surface roughness increased. The smoothest surface attainable, that obtained by using a jet of water and cleaning powder (Prophy-Jet), gave the highest bond strength, while the roughest surface gave the weakest.

The strongest bonds that have been reported in the literature are for the cement Chem-Fil and are 9.9 Mpa to enamel (citric acid) and 7.2 Mpa to dentine (Prophy-Jet treatment). The next highest are for ASPA IV: 7.5 Mpa to enamel (fluoride-containing surface cleaner) and 6.8 Mpa to dentine (25% poly(acrylic acid) treatment).

Bonding composite resins to glass-ionomer cements :

The use of glass-ionomer cements for replacement of carious dentine prior to attachment of composite resins to acid etched enamel was first described by McLean and Wilson (1977a). This work has resulted in the widespread use of glass-ionomer cements in the so-called "sandwich" or "double-laminated" technique, in which both cement and enamel are etched prior to attachment of a light-cured composite resin. This technique improves the bonding between the glass-ionomer cement and the composite resin. Overall, the laminate restoration has reduced microleakage compared with the simple composite resin restoration. These conclusions are supported by the findings of numerous research workers (McLean et al., 1985; Sneed and Looper, 1885; Welsh and Hembree, 1985; Gordon et al., 1985, 1986; Hinoura et al., 1987; Nara and Dogon, 1987).

Clinical applications of the sandwich technique have been reported by an increasing number of workers (Bitter, 1986; Garcia-Godoy and Malone, 1986). In the sandwich technique a glass-inomer cement is packed into the bottom of cavity, in effect to replace the lost dentine, and allowed to set and harden. When it has hardened it is acid etched (for up to one minute) using phosphoric acid solutions (37% aqueous). This treatment results in a rough surface in which glass particles stand proud of the matrix. Suitable for mechanical keying. A thin liquid dimethacrylate resin is then applied that penetrates into the interstices between the proud particles. The composite resin is subsequently packed into the cavity.

Acid etching

Glass-ionomer cements are appropriate for restoring cavities such as abrasion or erosion cavities where little or no cavity preparation is required. The tooth is, however, coated with a pellicle and other surface debris, so some sort of cleaning or conditioning treatment is required. The use of acid etchants with glass-ionomer cements has been advocated for many years. As the adhesion to tooth tissue is primarily mediated by the mineral component, the use of strong acids cause exposure of a collagen network in the dentin and a reduced bonding potential. Strong acids have been investigated extensively with the resin-based adhesive systems. Polyacrylic acid has a minor effect on the dentin, removing the smear layer and surface contaminants without opening the dentin tubules too widely. It has therefore become the etchant of choice for conventional glass-ionomers. There are two advantages in using polyacrylic acid for etching the dentin. First, because it is the acid used in the cement itself, any residue inadvertently left behind does not interfere with the setting reaction. Second, it enhances the wettability of the tooth surface to a water-containing cement and preactivates the calcium and phosphate ions in the dentin, rendering them more available for ion exchange with the cement·

Enamel bonding

The conventional glass-ionomer cements have very different interfacial characteristics with tooth tissue compared to those of resin composites and dentin bonding agents. As previously outlined, their adhesive mechanisms are restricted essentially to surface attraction. This restriction has severe implications if the materials become dimensionally unstable, which may happen as a result of excess water uptake or desiccation. Drying problems are most pronounced in relation to enamel, where the cement is adherent to the surface alone and where dehydration first appears clinically.

Dehydration can happen quickly intraorally with the placement of a rubber dam, or during impression taking procedures: the first sign of drying in the cement is a chalky white appearance on its surface. There usually are cracks below the enamel surface from previous cutting operations, so any shrinkage of the cement on drying causes cohesive failure of the substrate. The bond between glass-ionomer and enamel is stronger than is often realized; indeed, it can be stronger than the bond between enamel prisms, especially when these are running parallel with the cavity surface. This form of enamel fracture can be observed readily in any test sample where the material has not been maintained in a sufficiently hydrated form. Examination of fracture surfaces with scanning electron microscopy (SEM) can make it difficult to delineate enamel from cement, a difference which is seen easily with fluorescent labels and confocal microscopy.

Dentin bonding

The inherent wetness of the dentin interface may reduce the strength of the matrix close to the tooth by effectively reducing the powder-liquid ratio of the water setting cements. Microcracks can often be seen in this region. The net result may be cohesive failure of the cement in this region; an observation frequently reported in the literature.

The arcading within the matrix indicates the stresses imparted to the interface by the fluorescent labeled cement "dehydrating" and shrinking on setting. The band of fluorescent dye within the dentin is characteristic of any of the acid-base cements; even phosphate cement. Following etching with polyacrylic acid, the tubular openings may be exposed, making it is possible to see 2- to 3μm-long plugs of glass-ionomer cement matrix occupying these openings, especially if the cement is labeled with 0.2μm -diameter titanium dioxide particles and a reflection image made with a confocal microscope, These plugs may impart some mechanical interlocking to the adhesive interface but are in no way equivalent to the long tags seen with resin-based dentin bonding agents (DBAs).

Resin-Modified Glass-Ionomer Cements

Lining materials

The resin-modified cements were first introduced as lining materials, being unsuitable as restorative materials because of the marked polymerization shrinkage imparted by their high resin content. This resin component can be encouraged to act in a manner similar to that of DBAs with the use of suitable conditioning/priming systems. The light-curing capabilities of these liners offer some advantages in terms of increased resistance to acid dissolution when used with the acid-etch composite "sandwich" technique, but the high resin content allows particularly severe polymerization shrinkage. The fact that the liners are normally placed as thin layers also makes them more prone to dehydration, in much the same way as conventional glass-ionomers.

Restorative materials

Development of resin-modified glass-ionomers into restorative materials produces an interesting mixture of properties. The use of conditioners or primers containing 2-hydroxyethylmethacrylate (HEMA) produces interfacial appearances very similar to those of resin composites when the latter are used in conjunction with a DBA, an effect first noted with resin-modified lining materials.

Dynamic interactions can still occur with these new materials after the initial set. Resin-modified glass-ionomer cements can be porous to pulpal fluids, as indicated by dye uptake in the interfacial region of the cement. Examination of many samples suggests that a nonparticulate, easily stained layer of solid material (< 30 μm thick) often forms between the bulk of the cement and the dentin within 24 hours. This layer only forms next to dentin tubules that communicate with the wet pulp cavity and has been observed with Fuji II LC, Fuji Bond LC, and Photac-Fil Quick. Its presence with Vitremer is less discernible and may be doubtful. It is particularly obvious when fluorescent labeled solutions are placed in the pulp cavity, but it is not simply a contraction gap in which fluid has accumulated.

The solid interfacial layer is superficial to the cavity surface and is not a function of the acid etchants used, being present in interfaces where the smear layer has been removed by the use of an air abrasive stream. When the cut sample surface is imaged, it is seen to be intact and solid, which would be the appearance detected with conventional imaging techniques such as radiographs and SEM. Long tags of resin infiltrating dentin tubules are not a characteristic feature of resin-modified glass-ionomer cements. The term absorption layer has been applied to this structur it may be important in the maintenance of the fit of the restoration to compensate for the contraction of the resin on polymerization. This feature may be a resin layer at the restoration interface that has taken up fluid and swelled. It is not seen on the free outer surface of the restoration when it is soaked in dye-containing solutions, nor is it associated with enamel or a desiccated dentin surface.

Adhesives

The absorption layer is particularly marked in materials with a high HEMA-resin content, such as Fuji Bond LC, where labeling with special dyes and two-photon confocal imaging have shown HEMA distribution and the associated absorption layer next to the tooth interface.[103] This type of material is marketed as a stress-relieving bonding system for composites, in which the interfacial stresses from a shrinking, polymerizing composite restoration are dissipated by a resin-modified glass-ionomer cement that sets or polymerizes at a slower rate. Time lapse studies of restoration-tooth interfaces conducted in this laboratory indicate that the mechanism to counteract the polymerization shrinkage of the composite is one of swelling and movement within the immature cement as it takes up fluid from the dentin.

Dehydration shrinkage is still present with resin-modified cements. This happens very quickly and, after a few minutes, considerable gaps can open up in immature cements.[36] When failure is seen adjacent to the dentin, it is often in the absorption layer, whereas restorations with enamel margins often fail with structural cohesive failure of the enamel in a manner similar to that of conventional glass-ionomers.

Polyacid-Modified Resin Composites

The development of the polyacid-modified resin composites, or compomers, effectively completes the transition from materials with a water-based setting reaction to those that are almost entirely resin based. In contrast to resin composites, these materials are designed to be water tolerant in that they are required to absorb water for the development of the acid-base setting reaction after polymerization of the light-cured resin. In conventional glass-ionomers, the availability of free water to bound water decreases as the material matures over a period of months. Polyacid-modified composites also show an increase in bound versus free water as they mature, giving some evidence that they may have a limited glass-ionomer-type setting reaction.

Despite some evidence of such setting reactions, there is no inherent adhesion of polyacid-modified composites to tooth tissue. It is essential, therefore, that an intermediary adhesive be applied to the tooth. Most of the adhesives that have been produced for use with polyacid-modified composites are of the self- etching variety, so as to simplify handling. The manufacturers claim that etching with phosphoric acid is unnecessary. The low pH of the adhesive is sufficient to remove the smear layer and produce a resin infiltration zone in dentin. However, penetration into the dentin tubules is considerably reduced when compared with the same adhesive applied following phosphoric acid etching of the dentin. The penetration of resin tags into the enamel also is greatly reduced. There is therefore a risk of failure in both dentin and enamel at these interfaces when roughness of the substrate surface and penetration of the adhesive is reduced. However, a counter argument states that a "self-contained" primer etchant system will give penetration of the resin only as far as the etchant effect. This has been shown with one of the commercial adhesives available, with which excellent sealing of the interface is produced.

Hybrid zone formation

The concept of hybridization and micro-mechanical interlocking has become a popular explanation for the adhesion of resin-based DBAs when used for attaching resin composites. It is considered the major mechanism of attachment for the fluid hydrophilic resins often carried in volatile solvents, which impregnate the etched dentin surface and mediate the bond for the polyacid- modified composites. Much of the popularity for this concept stems from the relative ease of imaging these tough resin-tooth interfaces using SEM and transmission electron microscopy (TEM). However, the infiltration achieved may be only partial, with unfilled spaces in the acid-etched dentin interfcice. High- vacuum imaging techniques, such as SEM and TEM, cause great difficulty for observing water-containing cements. Therefore, despite the availability of environmental SEM, the concept of a hybrid zone has seldom been applied to conventional glass-ionomers, because it is difficult to produce interfacial images that are not seriously affected by the dehydration artifact.

The ion exchange that probably occurs at the tooth interface with glass-ionomer cements certainly yields a region with intermediate properties of both materials so in those terms it is a hybrid zone. However, the mechanisms involved are undoubtedly more subtle, relating more closely to the adsorption and diffusion theories of adhesion mentioned earlier than to the relatively macroscopic mechanical retention effects seen with resin infiltration.

Interfacial fracture

The failure of an adhesive joint involves three possible mechanisms, which may or may not occur in combination: cohesive failure in the substrate, cohesive failure within the adhesive, and adhesive failure. It is possible to image interfacial fracture of adhesive systems subjected to shear bond testing. Conventional glass-ionomers show deformation of the cement as load is applied, with slow propagation of cracks and flaws until catastrophic failure which often leaves a thin layer of residual cement, the ion-enriched layer on the tooth substrate. Resin-modified cements also can show significant flexibility, but this is usually most apparent in the absorption layer, especially in cements designed to act as an adhesive system for composite restorations.

Much of the published literature on dental adhesives uses load testing to rank effectiveness. The difficulty of making comparisons between different test centers because of variable specimen geometries and test configurations is well known. Making comparisons between different classes of material also is problematic because tough materials such as resin composites may perform well in a simple shear bond test; conventional glass-ionomers seldom perform as well because of their inherent weakness, which leads to their cohesive failure under these conditions. However, conventional glass-ionomers have other desirable properties such as limited setting shrinkage, good elasticity, and the ability to show self-repair mechanisms once cracks have appeared within them, as reported by Watson et al. and Feilzer et al. All these factors help in the survival of restorations in the oral environment.

Resin-modified glass-ionomers exhibit greater bonding strengths than do conventional glass-ionomers in shear bond testing. Polyacid-modified composites perform in a manner similar to that of conventional composites, their bond strength being related mainly to the effectiveness of the DBA used rather than their inherent adhesive properties.

11.GLASS IONOMERS AND COMPOMERS IN PEDIATRIC DENTISTRY

Glass ionomers and compomers in pediatric dentistry

The controversy (especially in Germany and Sweden) over dental amalgam and its alleged adverse health effects due to the release of mercury, governmental restrictions on its use, and still growing demand of patients for esthetic dentistry have led to an increased use of alternative filling materials. In Germany, the federal health authorities (BGA and BfArM) ruied in 1992, that amalgam fillings should no longer be placed in children under 6years of age, for reasons of potential prophylactic health care. However, the guidelines of these authorities contradict numerous German and international professional dental organizations on several issues and are not verified by independent scientific investigations.

During recent years, other restorative materials such as casting alloys, glass-ionomer cements, and resin composites also have received criticism due to their alleged side effects. In general, many of these allegations have been made without any documented scientific evidence. Like all their drugs, a certain risk of potential side effects, or residual risk, can never be excluded. However, based on current knowledge, it must be emphasized that one of the recommended restorative materials, including amalgam, resin composites, presents an irresponsible risk for the patient, who is the focus of all dental practitioners and material researches. Except for allergic and lichenous reactions, none of the supposed side effects has been clinically diagnosed.

The letter of Consensus issued on July 1, 1997, by the German Federal Ministry of Health, together with BfArM, the German Dental Association (BZAK/KZBV), the German Scientific Dental Association for Operative Dentistry (DGZ), satiates clearly that the stipulation of a general ranking of restorative materials is not justified based on current knowledge. In all cases, the decision about which restorative material is selected and used has to consider the clinical situation of the individual patient. Benefits and drawbacks of all possible restoratives materials must be estimated, and the informed patient needs to be involved in the treatment decision.

Glass-Ionomer and Resin Composite Restoratives

During the last two decades, many new filling materials and groups have been developed. The number of available restoratives has increased dramatically, especially during the last 5 years. The great variety of products originally made it difficult to classify the materials and caused uncertainty for dentists in identifying proper usage.

To create a clearly structured classification for tooth-colored plastic restorative materials, Hicket suggested assigning the materials to classes corresponding to their water content or a possible acid base reaction during setting. Consequently, two main groups were recognized glass-ionomer cements and resin composites with subdivision in each. Today, tooth-colored direct restorative materials are subdivided into the following groups: conventional and highly viscous glass-ionomer cements: resin modified glass-ionomer cements, or hybrid ionomers: and (hybrid and microfilled) resin composites, including dentin adhesive systems. Numerous products are available in each of these subgroups.

Conventional glass-ionomer cements

Conventional glass-ionomer materials represent the oldest category of glass-ionomers. They were developed during the late 1960s by Wilson and Kent.[2] The first commercial product, called ASPA, was introduced in 1972, and early materials required multiple improvements before gaining popularity in the 1980s. Changes were made in the glass particles, as well as in the composition of the polyacrylic acids. An essential improvement was the acceleration of the setting process, resulting in reduced moisture sensitively during the critical initial reaction period.

Metal-reinforced glass-ionomer cements

This type of cement is commonly referred to as cermet, derived from the abbreviation of ceramic and metal, or metal-modified glass-ionomer cement. Cermets were developed in the mid-1980s based on conventional glass-ionomers. Through high temperature sintering of silver particles to fusing glass powder, the wear resistance and flexural strength of the glass-ionomer cement was improved.

Precious to this development, efforts had been made to improve the properties of conventional cements by mixing alloy powder with the glass-ionomer powder: the resulting product was called Miracle Mix Metal-reinforced glass-ionomers show excellent radiopacity. However, they are not tooth-colored due to the addition of metal particles. In some cases, discoloration of restored teeth by oxidized silver particles has been reported. The bond strength to hard tooth tissues and the fluoride release of these materials are lower than those of conventional glass-ionomers.

Cermets are only available with silver particles (eg, Ketac-Silver, Chelon-Silver); versions with gold particles are not commercially available because of the high costs. Cemtents fell short of MccLean's high expectations as an alternative material to amalgam and exhibited frequent fractures in Class II cavities, as conventional glass-ionomer cements.

Highly viscous glass-ionomer cements

Due to the possibility of reduced secondary caries by fluoride release and to their comparative ease of use of conventional glass-ionomers, further developments have been made for posterior restoration in primary and permanent dentition. These highly viscous glass-ionomer cements are currently used in developing countries, in particular within the scope of atraumatic restorative treatment (ART) supported by the World Health Organization. The objective was to design a restorative material that be used without modern technical devices such as light-curing units, amalgamators, and micrometers that require electricity. Furthermore, a material with a high level of fluoride release was required because caries removal with hand instruments (eg, spoon excavators and enamel hatchets) is often incomplete, increasing the risk of recurrent caries or the development of new caries due to imperfect cavity margins.

The highly viscous glass-ionomer cements have been well accepted, especially in improved encapsulated versions (eg, Fuji IX GP, ketac-Molar). Due to their opacity, they have esthetic disadvantages when used for cervical fillings of Class III cavities. Predominant indications are filling in deciduous molars and temporary restorations in permanent posterior teeth.

The formulations of conventional, metal-reinforced, and highly viscous glass-ionomer cements have no additional functional polymerizable monomers. These cements are therefore advantageous for patients who are allergic to components of resin composites. Based on reports from Scandinavia, increasing rates of allergic reactions to monomers may be important for the future of these materials.

Resin-modified glass-ionomer cements

In the late 1970s and early 1980, the spread of light polymerization units began with the introduction of photopolymerizable resin composites. These materials became popular within a short time because of their handling and storage advantages. Light-curable glass-ionomers were developed in the mid-1980s, and are better described as hybrid ionomers or resin- modified glass-ionomers. Setting reaction of these materials has a light curing mechanism in addition to the acid base reaction of the glass-ionomer. The initial setting is by light-mediated polymerization of methacrylate monomers, while the slow acid-base reaction allows the bulk of the cement to mature to its final strength.

Most of the mechanical properties of hybrid ionomers (eg, flexural strength) are improved by the addition of the polymerizable monomers. The fluoride release rate of the resin-modified material is similar to that of conventional glass-ionomers; for patients with high levels of caries activity, both groups of materials may exhibit equivalent benefits. In spite of the resin content, wear resistance is low in most hybrid ionomers.

Due the usefulness of light polymerization, many dentists changed from conventional resin–modified glass-ionomers. Besides their ease of handling, they also offer reduced susceptibility to crazing and cracking as a result of desiccation. In deep cavities, light-cured materials can be completely polymerized only in thin increments (1.5 to 2 mm). Even in those areas of the mouth with limited access, the tip of the polymerization unit has to be placed as close to the restorative material as possible to obtain sufficient light intensity for the initial setting process.

Poly acid-modified resins and compomers

The term polyacid - modified resins was suggested by McLean et al. Unlike conventional and resin-modified glass ionomers, polyacid-modified resins and compomers have no or insignificant acid-base reaction during their setting process. Due to water sorption of the filling during clinical service, a negligible acid-base reaction can occur. Polyacid-modified resins are closely related chemically to compomers, which are sometimes integrated into this group. However, components, whereas polyacid modified resins are mixed with a precise powder-liquid ratio. Since the introduction of compomers, which offer easier handing, the importance of mixable polyacid-modified resins has significantly decreased.

The term compomer is derived from composite and glass-ionomer. This class of restorative materials combines some of the chemical and mechanical properties of resin composites with others of glass-ionomer cements. Compomers were introduced in the European market in 1993. Today, several products from different manufacturers are available. Compomers are similar to resin composites in their chemical structure. However, they include reactive, ion–leachable glass particles and polymerizable acidic monomers. In contrast to glass-ionomers, compomers contain no water in their formulations and are one-component materials, with the exception of dual curing compomers for cementation, which do not need mixing. An acid-base reaction, which is typical in the setting of glass-ionomer cements, does not occur during the setting process of compomers. However, similar to glass-ionomers, Compomers release fluoride[100].

With regard to their mechanical properties, particularly tensile and flexural strength and wear resistance, compomers are superior to glass-ionomers but less effective than resin composites. Prior to the application of compomer, the enamel and dentin need to be primed by bonding agent (acid etched) to obtain optimum adhesion and bond strength to hard tooth tissues. Glass-ionomer cements bond chemically to the tooth structure, partially by chelation of the calcium in the apatite to enamel and dentin with the carboxyl groups of their polyacids. In contrast, compomer bonding to tooth structure is primarily mediated by micromechanical retention (resin tags and resin–dentin-interdiffusion zone hybrid layer), as with resin composites.

Concerning esthetics and finishing polishing procedures, compomers are superior to conventional and even resin-modified glass-ionomer cements, although considerable differences may be found among individual products in all groups. They match almost perfectly with the surrounding tooth structure, unlike glass-ionomers, which sometimes look chalky and opaque.

Indications for Use

Until a few years ago, amalgam was the worldwide material of choice for the restoration of deciduous molars. However, a partial change has occurred due to the controversy over amalgam's possible side effects. Although Chistensen et al found that 73% of fillings were still amalgam, compared to glass ionomers (15%) and composite resins(10%). Widstrim and Forss[40] reported that in Finland amalgam fillings are inserted in only 29% of all adult patients and 15% of children and adolescents; glass-ionomer cements were used adolescents; glass-ionomer cements were used in 91% of restorations of primary teeth and in 47% of permanent teeth for patients up to 16 years of age. This frequency of glass-ionomer fillings is remarkably high in composition to other countries and depends greatly on the size and the locations. As shown in Table 11-3, conventional glass ionomers and cermets fracture more frequently in Class II cavities due to the comparatively low flexural strength of these materials. Olden burg et al reported 18% failure for Class II composite restorations in deciduous teeth, only 4% in Class I, and none in Class V lesions.

Therefore, indications for the different types of glass-ionomer cements and compomers are to some extent dependent on the type and size of the cavity. Due to a greater supply of better alternatives, conventional glass-ionomers are today mainly used in Class V and Class III cavities, especially for patients especially for patients exhibiting high caries activity. These materials also are employed for lesions in sclerotic dentin. Highly viscous glass-ionomer cements are esthetically inferior to all other types or materials described due to their high opacity. Except for the ART, they are applied only in deciduous molars and as temporary restorations in permanent posterior teeth.

Indications for resin–modified glass-ionomers correspond closely to those of conventional glass-ionomers; that is, primary indications are the restoration of cervical defects. They also are recommended for Class III cavities as well as for fillings in deciduous teeth.

Further developments, improvements, and clinical trials are needed to extend the indications for compomers to permanent restoration in Class I and Class II cavities in permanent dentition.

One important advantage of glass-ionomer cements is the release of fluoride. Hicks et al showed less formation of secondary cavities around glass-ionomers restorations in vitro. Svanberg et al reported less plaque formation on glass ionomers than on amalgam or resin composites. Caries-inhibiting effects also were described in a 5year in vivo study, and for pit and fissure sealants. In contrast, two articles about the reasons for replacement of failed restoration reported as high rate of secondary caries with glass-ionomer cements.

Considerably less fluoride is released from compomers than from resin-modified or conventional glass-ionomers. However, improvements have been made in this area and are still ongoing. For example amine fluoride has been added to the new primer systems and the percentage of fluoride-containing filler particles in compomers has been increased.

Clinical Procedures

Morphologic consideration of primary teeth

The technique of cavity preparation in primary dentition differs in part from that in permanent teeth. Several anatomic differences of primary teeth must be considered. Primary teeth have a thinner enamel (about 1 mm thick throughout the entire crown) than permanent teeth, and the distance occlusally and particularly mesiodistally from the tooth surface to the pulp chamber of the relative thickness of enamel and dentin is important in cavity preparation to avoid accidental pulp exposure. The pulp horns in primary teeth, especially the mesiobuccal pulp horn of the first deciduous molars, are high and prominent. Pulp chambers are proportionately larger; thus, there is comparatively less tooth structure protecting the pulp in primary teeth. The occlusal surface of primary molars is narrow, and the buccal and lingual surfaces diverge strongly towards the root, making the crowns rounded and bulbous. The distinct constriction at the neck of primary molars demands special care during preparation of the gingival seat of a proximal box. In contrast to permanent teeth, the orientation of the enamel rods of the gingival third of the crowns is directed toward the occlusal surfaces.

The mineral content of the enamel of primary teeth is lower than that of permanent dentition. Primary teeth show about 10 times more pores (1 to 5 vol%). In many cases, the enamel surface is characterized by a prismless outer layer, which is normally 30 to 50 μm thick but may be up to 100 μm. Due to this prismless layer, it was frequently postulated that adhesive composite restorations were not possible in deciduous teeth. However, when the enamel margins exposed, allowing adhesive bonded fillings even in primary teeth. The etching time was originally controversial in the past, 60-seconds etching of the enamel with 37% phosphoric acid was used for permanent teeth, and from 120 to 240 seconds was allowed for primary teeth. However, from 30 to 60 seconds, depending on the fluoride content of the enamel for deciduous teeth, is now considered sufficient to expose a proper microretentive etching pattern.[126,127]

Use of rubber dam

With few exceptions, the use of rubber dam in restorative pediatric dentistry is strongly recommended, regardless of the fillings materials. The isolation of the operating field presents many advantages, such as keeping spray from the dental handpiece, distasteful medicaments, disinfectants, monomers, and etching gel away from the tongue, throat, and soft tissues. It also saves time through elimination of spitting and rinsing by the patient, resulting in rare defensive reactions from the child. Tongue and lips are retracted and some what protected from rotating instruments. Many procedures in pediatric dentistry are performed more quickly and are less stressful when rubber dam is applied. This more than compensates for the short time required to place it.

Preparation and restoration

The formerly justified claims of "extension for prevention" have changed to "prevention of extension", thanks to highly improved preparation instruments and restorative materials and more sophisticated application techniques. Furthermore, high standards of oral hygiene and the availability of efficient mechanical devices and chemical agents for tooth cleaning and plaque removal are now available. Broader knowledge about the importance of proper dietary habits also has been achieved.

When employing adhesive restoratives, in contrast to amalgam fillings, unsupported but nonverbal enamel overhangs can be preserved and the cavity size can be kept as small as possible. The size of the cavity is mainly influenced by the extent of decay rather than by macroretentive considerations. Adhesive techniques result in the maximum preservation of tooth tissue, with positive effects on the strength and fracture restored tooth and filling.

After preparation of the primary outline form of the cavity and caries excavation, the margins are finished by smoothing with very fine diamond burs 25 μm grain size. Unlike cavities in anterior teeth, Class I and Class II cavities in primary teeth do not require specific beveling of the margins. This only enlarges the occlusal surface of the restoration unnecessarily. Internal and external line and point angles should be well rounded to permit better adaptation of the restorative material and adaptation of the restorative material and to lower stress concentration in the restoration and tooth reducing the potential for fractures.

Cervical lesions in deciduous dentition are rare and, in most cases, Completely limited to the enamel. If conventional glass-ionomer cements are used for restoring these cavities, butt joint margins are generally recommended to avoid fillings. On the other hand, if compomers or resin-modified Ionomers are employed. The margins can be prepared using a butt joint relationship between the tooth and the restorative material or by beveling.

With regard to compomers, there is still ongoing controversy about the necessity and usefulness of additional acid etching of the enamel margins. Acid etching results in a significantly higher bond strength of compomers to enamel. If the coronal margin in mixed Class V cavities is beveled and etched, the marginal quality is improved and there is less microleakage of compomer restorations in this area. However, in most cases, the gingival margin shows more marginal gaps in primed dentin due to the better and more durable adhesion and higher bond strength achieved with etched and primed enamel. An ideal solution for this problems is still pending.

In occlusal cavities of permanent molars, etching of the enamel improves the marginal quality, but no studies on primary teeth are available. At the present time, treatment in routine dental practice mainly occurs without additional etching because ease of use and time saved is a major benefit in treatment of children. All available studies have been carried out in compliance with this procedure.

In contrast to amalgam and resin composite restoration without the use of dentin adhesives, the application of a base or liner in deciduous teeth is not imperative for any of the restorative materials mentioned. Usually, due to limited cavity size, it is only recommended in deep cavities.

Acid etching of the tooth structures prior to filling should always be handled in compliance with the manufacture's instructions. Many glass-ionomers require etching of the dentin (eg, with 10% polycrylic acid) to remove the smear layer, thus improving the adhesion. Compomers must always be applied with the corresponding primer system.

When restoring Class II cavities, a matrix and wedges are placed prior to filling. The use of metal matrix bands, which are more reliable in producing physiologically controured proximal contact areas than plastic matrices, is approved for all Materials. Precontoured clear plastic matrices are available for Class V defects.

Conventional glass-ionomer cements can be bulk packed into the cavities witih a hand instrument or injected from a capule. Injected versions of glass ionomers are advantageous because they optimize the mixing process, have an ideal pre measured powder-liquied ratio, and facilitate placement into the cavity by direct injection. It is important to pay attention to the working time. If exceeded, it compromises the adhesive bond to tooth structure (accomplished by a chelation reaction between positively charged calcium ions present on the dentin and enamel surface, and setting by cross-linking chains of polyacrylic acids of the glass ionomer cements that contain negetively charged carboxyl groups).

Due to their moisture sensitivity, the surface of glass ionomer cements should be protected immediately at placement and during the intial setting stages. This can be accomplished with a special vernish (eg, Ketac Glaze) or a light cure-bonding agent to avoid desiccation or water uptake. Additional water sorption causes dissolution in the matrix and yields weaker cement with higher solubility. Dehydration results in crazing and cracking of the cement surface. Resin-modified glass-ionomers are less sensitive to moisture: however, their desiccation also results in a cracked and crazed surface. Therefore, these materials also should receive surface protection.

Although the resin-modified materials are dual-cured due to the acid-base reaction, attention should be given to sufficient light polymerzation. This is also imperative for compomers, which have to be applied increamentally in deep cavities, with each increment light cured individually for 40 seconds. This ensures proper polymerization with maximum material properties and significantly reduces shrinkage. Undercuring leads to a weakened restoration that is susceptible to failure during clinical service. The placement time for compomers is similar to that for amalgam.

Finishing and polishing

The process of contouring, finishing, and polishing resin-modified glass-ionomers, polyacid-modified resins, and compomers is basically equivalent to that for resin composite restorations. The anatomy of the occlusal surface should be shaped as much as possible with the appropriate hand instruments prior to polymerizatin. Flash material can be removed easily while compomer is still in a plastic condition. However, care must be taken not to compromise the marginal quality by removing excess material from the boundaries of the filling. Finishing and pollishing can be intiated immediately after polymerization. The margins of the restoration are smoothed with fine-grit finishing diamond burs, and the occlusal anatomy is improved. Occlusal contacts and lateral movement paths are contrlled and refined, if needed. Polishing is done with flexible aluminum oxide disks, abrasive silicon points, and cups provided by different manufactures. A final high-gloss appearance can be achieved with fine and extra-fine composiite polishing pastes applied with mandriel-mounted foam polishing cups.

For conventional glass-ionomers, the following finishing and polishing procedure has proven successful. Depending on the product, approximately 5 minutes after placement of the glass-ionmer into the cavity, the matrix is removed and the excess cement at the margins is trimmed without water spray using hand instruments. It is important that all carving is done from the restoration toward the hard tooth tissue and not in reverse, to avoid ditching of the cement at the margins. After removal of the flash, the surface of the glass-ionomer restoration is coated with a protective varnish/ bonding agent to avoid dehydration and water sorptin. Occlusion is checked for proper contact, if applicable. Further finishing and polishing should be done during the next appointment, ideally at least 24 hours later when the cement has reached its full maturity. Sufficient water-cooling during rotariy instrumentation is imperative. If the glass ionomer cement becomes heated because of dry instrumentation, cracking and crazing in the cement will occur due to desiccation. Ultrafine finishing diamonds (15 μm grain size) are used for contouring and finishing. Final polishing is accomplished with fine and ultrafine flexible abrasive aluminum oxide disks. Sufficient cooling with water spray is necessary throughout the entire process.

Clinical Results In Primary Dentition

In comparison to restorations in permanent dentition, the longevity of those in primary teeth is significantly diffirent for all materials. This makes the assessment of these fillings as a separate group meaningful. Qvist et al and others found an average longevity of less than 2 years for amalgam fillings in children 4 years old and under, and only 1 year or less for composite restorations in this age group. According holland et al failure of amalgam fillings occurs more frequently in decidous teeth, especially in small children, due to moisture contamination of the cavities during condensation. The age of the children at the time of placement is therefore a major factor in restoration longevity.

In contrast to studies of permanent dentition, no separate investigations of glass-ionomer fillings in Class III and Class V lesions in primary dentition are known for this reason, only Class I and Class II restorations in deciduous molars are discussed.

Studies of primary molars with resin composite and amalgam restorations have presented different results. Barr-Agholme et al reported significantly better results for composite restorations (88% satisfactory) after 2 years compared to amalgam (68%), while Ostlund et al found better results for amalgam fillings (92% acceptable) than for composites (84%) or glass ionomers (40%) after 3 years of service. Varpio revealed less favorable results with earlier resin composites, which had less than 60% success after 3 years and only abut 35% acceptability after 4 to 6 years. Oldenburg et al found a success rate of 89% after 4 years for composite restorations, but reported great discrepancies between different types of restorations.

Conventional and metal-reinforced glass-ionomer cements

During the last 10 to 20 Years, glass-ionomer cements have been employed to an increasing degree as a restorative material in the primary dentition.[66-70,86-93] walls et al[66] showed that after 2 years of clinical service the performance of glass-ionomer cements in posterior teeth was similar to that of amalgam fillings. But, after 5 years, amalgam had median survival time of 3.5 years, which was superior to that of conventional glass inomers (2.8 years). Qvist et al compared amalgam and conventinal glass-ionomer cements after 3 years and found a significantly higher failure rate with glass-ionomers, especially in Class II cavities. [95]

Cermet restorations revealed a comparable success rate to amalgam filling in small children. In older children and larger cavities, especially in Class II restorations, amalgam was superior. Compared to amalgam, encapsulated glass-ionomers offered the advantege of a shorter application time.[96]

Highly viscous glass-ionomer cements

Due to the relative newness of highly viscous glass-ionomers, only a few clinical studies using these materials in primary molars have been published. Franken berger et al reported a 72% success rate for Hi-Dense with an observatin period up to 2 years, showing no statistically significant difference compared to the results using Ketac-Silver. As in previous studies of conventional glass-ionomers and cermets, Hi-Dense revealed more factures in Class II cavities than in Class I lesions. This result was to be expected because of the low flexural strength of the resin-free glass-ionomer cements compared to resin-modified materials and compomers.[16, 17]

Resin-modified glass-ionomer cements

Few published studies are available for the hybrid ionomers. Kimura et al compared conventional glass-ionomers with resin-modified cements and found a higher success rate for the latter, with the same anticariogenic effect for both materials. The resin-modified material vitremer showed a better marginal adaptation than cermet, as observed by Espelid and Tveit. Donly et al reported equivalent results for resin-mdified cement and amalgam. Croll and Helpin analyzed more than 250 Vitremer Class II restorations after 12 to 18 months and observed no fractures, no marginal stain, no recurrent caries, and only minor wear.[171]

Compomers

With the introduction of compomers, the number of restorations in primary dentition using conventional glass-ionomers and cermet decreased dramamtically. The same was true for amalgam in Germany and some other European countries. Even through compomers represent the most recent class of material discussed, several studies with an observation period up to 3 Years exist. At present, compomers show the highest success rate of all materials in deciduous molars, more than 90% after 3 years (Tables 11-7 and 11-8). In many cases, compomers are the material of choice .

Clinical Results in Mixed Dentition

Restoration in permanent teeth of children show generally better results than those in primary teeth but still shorter longevity compared to adults, possibly due to lack of co-oporation during treatment. Fillings in permanent teeth of children and adolescents are intial restorations in most cases. This distinguishes them from those in adults, where approximately two thirds of restorations are caused by replacement of existing fillings due to failure. If caries is diagnosed early, intial restorations usually can be limited by preserving a maximum of sound tooth structure. This is possible thanks to modern and sophisticated diagnostic and preparation instruments, restorative materials, and application techniques, as well as to appropriate patient motivation and education in good oral hygiene.

With the introduction of Sonicsys, an ultrasonic-driven cavity preparation system, and modern restorative materials (such as low-viscosity light-curing resin composites, or flowable composites), It is possible to prepare even proximal minimally invasive cavities without advarsely touching the approximal tooth and to place adhesive restorations. Because small fillings are less stressed by chewing forces and show a greater longevity, maximum preservation and protection of natural tooth tissue should still gain in importance in the future.[17, 91, 95]

Summary

In spite substantial improvements during the 1980s, conventional glass-ionomer cements still have shortcomings with regard to moisture sensitvity; wear resistance, flexural strength, and final polishing. Even though the chemical adhesion to enamel and dentin and the fluoride release are major benefits, conventional glass-ionomers are restricted to special indications (Class III and Class V cavities) in operative dentistry.

The use of conventional glass-ionomer cements and metal-reinforced cements has decreased due to the development of new restorative materials; such has highly viscous glass-ionomers and compomers. However, conventional glass-inomer cements are still an important alternative filling material for patients suffering from allergies to polymerizable resin monomers.

Resin–modified glass-ionoimer and cements cover the same indications as conventional glass-ionomers. Both materials have a low resistance to abrasion. Therefore, they should not be employed in stress-bearing areas in posterior teeth. To what extent the more wear-resistant highly viscous glass-ionomers and compomers can be used in these areas, with or without limitations reading cavity size is a crucial factor in the planning of future controlled clinical trials.

Given improved measures in oral prophylaxis, significantly fewer and smaller cavitites will be found in children and adolescents in the future. These lesions probably will be indicated for filling materials that are currently not qualified for large stress-bearing restorations. In primary dentition, compomers, resin-mdified glass-ionomers, and highly viscous glass-ionomers, are excellent alternative filling materials.

Sealants and preventive restorations

Glass-ionomer materials have been suggested for fissure sealing, although there is relatively limited evidence as to the effectiveness of this technique. Results of a study by McLean and Wilson showed 78% retention of glass-ionomer fissure sealants after 2 years, but others have reported a total or substantial loss of sealants after 6 months. It may be relevant that Mclean and Wilson recommended that glass-ionomer cements be used only on fissures that were wider than 100 μ.

An extension of the sealant procedure may be the use of glass ionomers in the restoration of occlusally protected or small-access occlusal cavities, with the application of a resin-based fissure sealant to the glass-ionomer surface and remaining fissures. Such a restoration has been termed a "preventive glass-ionomer restoration" by Garcia-Godoy. If radiographic examination of the tooth indicates that the extent of carious attack is limited to the outer third of the dentin and examination of the occlusion reveals a lack of occlusal contact with the proposed restoration, the technique may be considered.

Caries may be removed with a small round bur or with other ultraconservative cavity preparation methods. The glass-ionomer is applied to the cavity and, when set, the enamel margins of the cavity and the fissures are etched as appropriate. The tooth is rinsed and dried and the sealant applied and cured. The occlusion should be checked and adjusted as necessary; sealant should be reapplied to any areas of glass-ionomer that have been exposed during adjustment. It is desirable for the type of glass-ionomer material chosen for this application to be among the most wear resistant available; cermets, or metal- reinforced materials, may therefore be most appropriate. Such restorations may from time to time be resurfaced or converted to a sandwich restoration.

Occlusal restorations

Early glass-ionomer materials lacked the physical properties of high tensile strength and wear resistance necessary for use in Class I situations. Metal-reinforced glass-ionomer cements were initially considered promising as an alternative to dental amalgam in such situations, but failed to gain popularity or to demonstrate effectiveness in this application. Newer, more heavily filled glass-ionomers may possess improved wear resistance. The tensile strength of these materials also is sufficiently improved to permit their evaluation in Class I cavities in limited situations such as the following:

- In small to medium-sized restorations that are protected from occlusal forces by remaining tooth structure
- For patients with a perceived need for fluoride release
- For patients who request a tooth-colored restoration and are prepared to accept a long-term provisional restoration, which may be placed at a lower cost than other tooth-colored restorations such as resin composite
- For nervous, phobic patients in whom the use of materials that require more time to place or are technique sensitive may be precluded
- When an easy-to-place restoration is required, as in atraumatic restorative treatment
- When the margins of large load bearing restorations require repair

Preparation for occlusal glass-ionomer restorations should first involve careful examination of occlusal contacts, with the occlusal outline being prepared to avoid such contacts if possible. Margins should not be beveled, because this may leave a thin flash of glass-ionomer material that may fracture during function. Following finishing of the restoration, the surface should be cleaned and sealed with a layer of unfilled resin; this may form part of a preventive approach by sealing the remaining fissures. There is an urgent need to evaluate the performance of contemporary glass-ionomer restorations in Class I cavities and to assess the cost-effectiveness of such restorations.

Tunnel restorations

The tunnel restoration was first described by Jinks in 1963 as a conservative alternative to the conventional procedure for Class II cavity preparation in primary molars. He suggested that, following preparation of a Class I lesion in an occlusal fossa, a small round bur could be used to prepare a "tunnel" diagonally under the marginal ridge and into the primary caries. Jinks, who originally suggested the use of a sodium silica-fluoride cement containing silver alloy filings, abandoned tunnel restorations because of a marginal ridge fracture rate of between 12% and 15%.

With the introduction of glass-ionomer materials, tunnel restorations have enjoyed renewed interest, with Hunt, Knight, and McLean independently suggesting the use of glass-ionomers in tunnel restorations in deciduous and permanent teeth. In this application, the glass-ionomer cement is syringed into the proximal lesion prior to the restoration of the occlusal access cavity with a resin- based material.

With regard to the performance of tunnel restorations, Croll did not report any cases of marginal ridge fracture or recurrent caries in "dozens" of cases, and the consensus view from laboratory experiments is that the strength of the marginal ridge of teeth restored with tunnel cermet restorations is as great as that of unrestored sound teeth or at least as that of teeth restored with composite. Lumley and Fisher, however, have published data on a long-term pilot study of tunnel restorations stating that 25% of glass-ionomer and 10% of cermet tunnel restorations failed, whereas none of the small Class II amalgam restorations placed as controls required replacement. In a study of tunnel restorations in 27 children, Zenkner and coworkers demonstrated that caries was not eliminated in a large proportion of cases, although the long-term significance of this was not elucidated.

The use of magnification techniques may be considered essential for carrying out tunnel restorations. Caries detection solutions also may be helpful in ensuring complete removal of the lesion. It is suggested that tunnel restorations are most successfully completed when they are prepared using an intraoral video camera in conjunction with a lens that permits accurate viewing of the operative field.

The advantages of the tunnel technique are retention of the marginal ridge and interproximal contacts; disadvantages include the difficulty in locating proximal caries and ensuring its removal. Anecdotal evidence also indicates that practitioners consider tunnel restorations difficult to complete with confidence. For these reasons, the tunnel restoration has not achieved great popularity, as confirmed by statistics provided by the National Health Service in the United Kingdom. These results showed that only 10,538 tunnel restorations were placed in 1 year, compared to 4.7 million Class II amalgam restorations, although more than half of the latter may have been replacements of defective restorations. The failure of the few clinical evaluations carried out to demonstrate the advantages of tunnel restorations over Class II amalgam and resin composite restoralions in permanent teeth tend to indicate that the clinical acceptance of this technique will continue to be limited, at least in the foreseeable future.[124, 137]

An alternative approach to the operative management of small proximal carious lesions may be the "lateral" tunnel, or slot, preparation described by Morand and Jonas and using either a bur or newer ultrasonic means of preparation. In this technique, the proximal lesion is accessed from the lingual or buccal surface, with the preservation of substantial amounts of tooth tissue, including the marginal ridge. Optical aids and fiber-optic illumination are required to view the lesion and its preparation. This technique may be particularly useful for elderly patients who have suffered gingival recession which thereby facilitate access to the lesion. As with the tunnel concept, a radiopaque glass ionomer is most appropriate, so the proximal area may be checked radiographically for recurrent caries. Morand and Jonas have provided guidelines for the success of such preparations. These include the removal of the smear layer prior to application of a resin-modified glass-ionomer, placement of the material using a syringe to avoid incorporation of air bubbles or voids, and tight compression of the matrix. As with the use of glass-ionomers in Class I situations, randomized clinical trials are required to investigate the long-term efficacy of lateral tunnel restorations.[98]

Atraumatic restorative treatment

In developing countries, most dental caries is left untreated and, if treated, is managed by extraction. Reasons for the lack of treatment may include the remote locations of the population; inadequate number and distribution of dental personnel; lack of availability of reliable water supplies; and insufficient finances to purchase equipment, materials, the services of oral health professionals, and the premises in which they may operate (if only a mobile surgery unit). Furthermore, most restorative dentistry carried out in industrialized countries is highly dependent on the availability of suitable electrically powered equipment. However, electricity is neither available nor reliable in rural or suburban areas of many less industrialized countries, and contemporary dental procedures are therefore difficult to carry out. As a result, the inhabitants of such countries may not benefit from recent developments in dental materials and techniques.

The atraumatic restorative treatment (ART) was first evaluated in Tanzania in; the mid-1980s, along with interested manufacturers of materials, based on manual excavation of caries and the use of an adhesive restorative material and sealant (currently, but not originally, a reinforced glass-ionomer). This makes it an appropriate intervention for people living in underdeveloped countries, other groups such as refugees, and people living in deprived communities who are unable to obtain restorative dental care. This technique, however, is only one component of oral health care that also must include promotion of other messages such as a nutritionally balanced diet, good oral hygiene, and the use of a fluoride-containing toothpaste.

The ART concept need not be confined to less industrialized countries. Because it is based on the concept of minimal intervention and minimal cavity preparation, there is potential for its application in restorative treatment in children. It also may provide a treatment option for groups such as the physically or mentally handicapped, persons living in shelters, and those receiving home care services.

With regard to the success of the technique, results of a study on the longevity of restorations placed under field conditions in rural Thailand using ART with glass-ionomer restorations, based on evaluation criteria that included the absence or presence of restorations and of marginal defects, indicated that the success rate of single-surface restorations in permanent teeth was 93% and 67% for dual-surface restorations after 1 year; in deciduous teeth, the success rates were 79% and 55% for single-surface and dual-surface restorations, respectively. Results of a study in Zimbabwe indicated that 85% of single-surface restorations in permanent teeth were rated good or acceptable after 3 years, and ART has been well received by the majority of patients.

The principal stages in the ART technique are isolating the tooth with cotton rolls, cleaning it with wet cotton pellets, obtaining access to the carious lesion with a hatchet or similar instrument, removing the soft carious material with an excavator, providing pulpal protection if necessary, and placing the restorative material. The occlusion should be checked, any excess material removed before it has hardened, and the res- toration coated with varnish or petroleum jelly. Limitations to ART include hand fatigue during instrumentation. The technique takes no less time than an amalgam restoration and works best on minimal cavities in permanent teeth. To allow the glass-ionomer to perform optimally, there must be sufficient tooth substance to surround the restoration. There are no long-term clinical data on its success.

The size of the lesion appears to be of particular importance. Atraumatic restorative treatment is most appropriate to small cavities, because, with the limited treatment availability in such situations, the best treatment of large carious lesions may be to render the cavity self-cleansing in the hope that the caries will be arrested. However, access to a minimal lesion may be difficult without a drill.

Sandwich restorations

It has been shown that it is possible to bond resin composite materials to glass- ionomer cements. Given that glass-ionomer cements bond to both enamel and dentin, it also is possible to bond a resin composite restoration to dentin with an intermediate layer of glass-ionomer. This is known as a sandwich, or laminate, restoration. The sandwich restoration may be "open," when the glass-ionomer forms part of the external surface of the restoration, or "closed," when the glass-ionomer is completely contained by the overlying composite.

Initially, acid etching of the glass- ionomer surface was considered necessary to produce satisfactory bond strengths, but etching during the maturation phase of the cement was found by Taggart and Pearson to adversely affect the material. These researchers concluded, after a series of laboratory tests, that the practice of etching a glass-ionomer was not advisable, but that, if etching were considered, it should be carried out for no longer than 10 seconds and preferably 24 hours after mixing, which is not a clinically viable option.

In the sandwich restoration, a glass-ionomer cement is used to replace the dentin of the cavity, with a resin composite used in conjunction with acid etching of the enamel to provide an esthetic restoration of the remaining cavity. This technique may be applied to Class I, Class II, Class III, and Class V lesions, and the chemical bond and leaching of fluoride optimize the properties of the resin composite and the glass-ionomer.

The sandwich technique also may be employed for posterior restorations, using either an open or closed version. Results from a survey in Australia indicated that 65% of respondent dentists used this technique, but clinical observation of biological problems such as pulp symptoms and secondary caries were said to occur "often", with 14% of the respondents also reporting dissolution or wear of the proximal cement. Forsten et al reported similar results from a survey in Scandinavia, with wear or dissolution of the open proximal glass-ionomer cement surface being reported by 17% of respondents. Furthermore, results of a clinical trial using a similar technique, reported by Welbury and Murray, demonstrated the limitations of the technique; the authors concluded that the sandwich technique failed to provide acceptable restorations during their trial. It would therefore appear that the open sandwich technique is not to be recommended. However, the closed technique, using the glass-ionomer as a thick base to replace the dentin, appears to be well liked by operators, although no data are available on the long-term clinical success of the technique in posterior teeth.

Factors dictating the choice of glass-ionomer material for sandwich restorations include the mechanical stress to which the cement-resin union is to be subjected and the desirability of radiopacity in the cement. If mechanical stress is expected to be high, a cement with optimal compressive and tensile strengths should be used, along with a resin composite with low polymerization shrinkage and a bonding agent with high wettability. If the restoration is in a posterior tooth, a radioopaque cement such as a cermet or lining cement should be used.[101]

A clinical routine described by Mount suggests preparing the cavity without beveling, etching the entire cavity with 10% polyacrylic acid for 20 seconds and rinsing for 15 seconds, placing matrix and wedge, and inserting the glass-ionomer cement to cover the entire dentin, except at the gingival floor. The cement is trimmed to provide a flat gingival floor and axial wall and the excess removed from the enamel, which is etched with 35% phosphoric acid for 30 seconds and rinsed for 15 seconds. Unfilled resin is then applied to the cement and etched enamel. The composite restoration is then cured and finished.[101]

Core buildup

The construction of a core, or foundation restoration, is often necessary prior to crown preparation in order to give the final crown appropriate resistance and retention. By implication, the core should have its own retention by means of retentive features in the buildup cavity, pins or posts, or the use of a material that reliably adheres to tooth structure.

Following placement of a crown, the core becomes an integral part of the load bearing structure of the tooth; it is therefore essential that the mechanical properties of the core are adequate for this function. Among the properties a core buildup material should possess are adequate compressive, tensile, and flexural strengths; nonirritance to tooth tissue; radiopacity similar to that of enamel; a coefficient of thermal expansion similar to that of dentin; low thermal conductivity; the ability to adhere to or be bonded to tooth structure, pins, and/or posts; ease of mixing and placement; short setting time; lack of adverse reaction to temporary crown materials or cements; and a color that contrasts with that of the tooth.

Until recently, amalgam was thought to afford the most favorable physical characteristics for core buildup procedures. However, amalgam cannot be built up and prepared in one visit, nor does it adhere to tooth tissue unless amalgam-bonding techniques are employed. Early glass-ionomer materials lacked the necessary tensile and flexural strengths for anything other than fashioning small core buildups or blocking out undercuts in preparations, but the improved tensile strength and fracture toughness of resin-modified glass-ionomers and heavily filled glass-ionomers make these materials appropriate for core buildups. Further more, the coefficient of thermal expansion of these materials approximates that of tooth tissues more than resin composite does, and they therefore may possess many of the properties associated with the ideal core buildup material.

No currently available material appears to possess sufficient adhesion to tooth to permit its use without additional retention by means of pins, posts, or retentive features where there has been extensive loss of tooth tissue. Current thoughts on core buildups negate the use of pins and posts wherever possible, with the foundation material being packed into the pulp chamber in root-filled teeth. In vital teeth, it is essential that efforts be made to conserve all remaining tooth tissue during core buildup and subsequent preparation, including ferruling to limit damaging stresses.

Classification of Proximal Carious Cavities

Mount considered some modification of conventional cavity design appropriate for proximal lesions. These ideas have been further refined and developed, with Mount and Hume suggesting a new classification for cavities that may be particularly appropriate to accommodate the "new" caries situations, such as those seen in gerodontics. These include circumferential cavities at the gingival margin and proximal lesions that are inappropriate for conventional Class II restorations.

The suggested classification takes into account the site, size, and complexity of the lesion. Site 1 lesions are similar to Class I lesions, namely those originating in pits and fissures. Site 2 lesions are those associated with contact areas and are divided into subcategories: size 1 (minimal), size 2 (moderate), size 3 (enlarged), and size 4 (extensive). Site 3 lesions are those originating close to the gingival margin around the full circumference of a tooth. This would include those lesions referred to as Black's Class V lesions and includes cavities occurring on mesial or distal tooth surfaces following gingival recession. Site 2, size 1 (#2,1) lesions would therefore be appropriate for restoration by a tunnel, slot, or other minimal cavity preparation designed to maintain the maximum amount of tooth structure. Glass-ionomer cement may be considered an appropriate material for such cavities, and it therefore follows that this revised classification of carious lesions may be more appropriate to modern adhesive restoratives than the classification suggested by G. V. Black almost a century ago.

Improving the Performance of Glass-lonomer Materials

Glass-ionomer materials possess many beneficial characteristics. It would therefore be reasonable for manufacturers and researchers to attempt to overcome the negative characteristics in order to expand the indications for use, particularly in load-bearing situations. Increasing the powder-liquid ratio is one method by which the physical properties of glass-ionomer cements may be improved, with a consistency requirement similar to putty being suggested. Newer materials appear to fulfill this requirement, with their improved physical properties due in part to a reduction in size of the glass particles in the matrix. Some of these materials may be condensable, but not to the extent of amalgam. Correct handling of materials and pretreatment of dentin also are valuable in enhancing the properties of glass-ionomer materials, as are delayed finishing and protection of the restorations.

12.APPLICATION OF GLASS-IONOMER CEMENTS IN ENDODONTICS

Glass ionomer cements have been widely used in medicine, mainly in otologic and reconstructive surgery and orthopaedics. Because these cements produce no heat while setting, they will not cause thermal damage to tissue and will not affect heat-labile drugs incorporated in the matrix phase of the cement (Wilson and Mclean 1988, Wittwer et al. 1994). Unset GIC's bind to bone (apatite) and metals (Mclean 1988, Wilson & Mclean 1988) and do not undergo appreciable shrinkage while setting (Mclean 1988, Wilson & Mclean 1988,Hill et al. 1995). Their main use in medicine is the stabilization of implanted devices and bony fragments and reconstruction or obliteration of bony defects (Geyer & Helms 1990, Babhigian 1992, Geyer 1992, Ramsden et al. 1992, Muller et al 1993,1994, Mcelveen 1994).

Glass-ionomer cements have been used in endodontics for sealing root canals orthogradely and retrogradely, for sealing and restoring the pulp chamber, for repairing perforations, and rarely for treating vertically fractured teeth. These applications, which evolved in the 1980s and 1990s, share their rationale with the more common application of glass-ionomer cement as a restorative material and a luting cement. Thus glass-ionomer cement is used in endodontics for its capacity to bond to dentin, its good biocompatibility and its fluoride release. The first property is expected to enhance the seal and reinforce the tooth, the second to minimize the irritation of the periradicular tissues, and the third to impart an antimicrobial effect to combat root canal infection.

The use of GIC in root canals was first introduced by Pitt Ford (1979) in a laboratory study. Using a single cone technique (gutta-percha or silver cones in combination with a GIC), he found that woring time was too short to be used in conjunction with the lateral compaction technique. Stewert (1990) proposed two other formulations in order to prolong the working time, and added barium sulphate to increase radiopacity. Ray & Seltzer (1991) developed a usable experimental formulation with adequate working time, radiopacity and adhesion to the root canal wall. These modifications led to the commercialization of **Ketac-Endo** (ESPE, Seafeld, Germany) in 1991.

Apart from the conventionally hardening cements RMGIC's were also tested. Saunder's et al. (1992) tested Vitrebond in combination with gutta-percha and showed that there was good adaptation of the sealer to the canal

Good adhesion and a strong material contribute to the strength of the tooth. In an in vitro study, Trope & Ray (1992) found an increased resistance to certical fracture, when obturating canals in conjunction with a glass ionomer sealer.

More recent developments are two experimental GIC sealer formulations: **KT-308** (GC Corp, Tokyo, Japan; Lalh et al. 1999a), which is a conventional GIC with an increased radiopacity and an extended working time, and **'ZUT'** (University of Toranto, Canada, Lalh et al1999a), consisting of KT-308 combined with an antimicrobial agent, a silver-containing zeolite (0.2%-

20% weight) 'ZUT' demonstrated an effective suppression of adherent *Enterococcus faecalis* over a 12 week period (Patel et al 2000), which may promote its efficacy as a root canal sealer.

The proven clinical efficacy of GIC's in medical applications also suggests potential advantages for the field of surgical endodontics: minimal irritation of periradicular tissues may be expected and it is known that the fluoride release may contribute to bone Mineralization (Tencer's et al. 1989).

General properties – endodontic perspective

Root Canal Sealing

The outcome of root canal treatment critically depends on the elimination of existing root canal infection and the long-term prevention of reinfection. In many cases, the root canal cannot be disinfected predictably using conventional intracanal procedures. There may be an advantage, therefore, in filling the canal with materials that can eliminate or curtail the residual microorganisms. Such materials also may resist the ingress of microorganisms and prevent reinfection.

The root canal, being normally free of salivary or blood contamination, is an ideal environment for the placement of glass-ionomer cement. The concept of using this cement as a root canal sealer was first introduced by Pitt Ford. Using a commercially available restorative material in conjunction with silver cones, he observed that the material set too quickly to allow application in conjunction with condensed gutta-percha. To extend the working time, Stewart mixed together two formulations of glass-ionomer cement, then added barium sulfate to increase the radiopacity. Ray and Seltzer filled root canals entirely with a modified glass-ionomer cement and concluded that it was easy to use, was adequately radiopaque, and adapted closely to the canal wall. This material was later introduced commercially (Ketac-Endo), and to date it is the sole glass-ionomer cement available specifically as a root canal sealer. Similarly, Saunders et al used a resin-based glass-ionomer cement (Vitre-bond) as a root canal sealer in conjunction with gutta-percha and found it adapted closely to the canal wall. In addition, Trope and Rayg reported that roots filled with a glass-ionomer cement had an increased resistance to vertical fracture. All these early reports formed the basis for the use of glass-ionomer cement as a root canal sealer in endodontic therapy .

Retreatability and removal

Any material used for root canal filling has to allow retreatment of the canal. For this reason, the glass-ionomer cement sealer is placed in conjunction with a gutta-percha cone. Retreatment is facilitated by dissolving the gutta-percha and using ultrasonic vibration in the canal to disperse the cement. In a series of in vitro studies, glass-ionomer cement was slower to retreat than conventional sealers; however, it could be removed effectively without an excessive amount of residue attached to the canal walls. Partial removal of the root filling, for preparation of a post space, also is somewhat slower in canals filled with glass-ionomer cement than in those filled with other sealers.

Sealing efficacy

Since the introduction of glass-ionomer cement as a root canal sealer, its sealing efficacy has been the subject of many in vitro studies employing different methodologies. The results of these study are diverse and inconclusive, and their clinical relevance questionable. In a few studies, the seal provided by the glass-ionomer cement was poor however, in the majority it was comparable to the seal provided by conventional sealers are better. The seal may be improved by using the cement in conjunction with condensed gutta-percha rather than with a single gutta-percha cone, but this suggestion has been disputed. As with all other root canal sealers, the seal appears to be conversely related to the thickness of the sealer layer. Possibly, when applied in bulk, the shrinkage of the glass-ionomer cement undermines the seal of the root canal space.

Recently, Friedman et al introduced an animal model designed to assess the resistance of root fillings to bacterial ingress from an inoculated pulp chamber. Such evaluation closely simulates clinical conditions and is considered more relevant than evaluations in vitro. When tested with this model, an experimental glass-ionomer cement sealer performed better than a conventional sealer of a zinc oxide-eugenol type.

Antimicrobial efficacy

The antimicrobial activity of glass-ionomer cement is believed to result from the release of fluoride. The uptake of fluoride by the root canal dentin has been studied by Saunders et al. Using a resin-based glass-ionomer cement as a sealer, these researchers observed a variable degree of increase in fluoride in the dentin after periods of 2, 4, and 12 weeks.

Conventionally setting glass ionomer cements:

Several studies have addressed the potential antimicrobial efficacy of glass- ionomer cement sealers. In the agar diffusion test, two glass-ionomer cements demonstrated a strong antimicrobial effect when freshly mixed and after 48 hours. In this short time frame, the antimicrobial efficacy of these cements was better than that of several conventional sealers. In a direct contact test, the short-term antimicrobial efficacy of a glass-ionomer cement was comparable to that of a zinc-oxide-eugenol sealer; however, within 1 week it diminished considerably. In another study, an experimental glass-ionomer cement sealer failed to suppress the growth of microorganisms on its surface. In a model designed to assess the antimicrobial effect of materials within the dentinal tubules of bovine teeth, a glass- ionomer cement sealer had no effect within the first 24 hours· After 7 days, however, some antimicrobial effect was evident, although considerably less than that of other sealers.

Studies on the antibacterial activity of GICs related to theiruse in endodontics are few, although the bacterial inhibition of Ketac-Endo endodontic sealer has been reported. Abdulkader et al. (1996) found that Ketac-Endo inhibited all the bacteria usedin their study. The antimicrobial action, according to the authors, was related to the low pH, when freshly prepared (Mount 1994), and the potential to release fluoride ions (Tobias et al. 1985, Meryon & Johnson 1989). The possibility that other components were involved was not excluded. Heling & Chandler (1996) found antibacterial activity only after 7 days for Ketac-Endo and none at 24 hr. in another study; Shalhav et al. (1997) concluded that Ketac-Endo possessed a very potent but short-acting antibacterial activity.

Two experimental GIC root canal sealers ('KT-308' and 'ZUT') were tested in different studies for antibacterial activity against E.faecalis. Depending on the experimental design, different results were obtained. 'ZUT' demonstrated a significant reduction in bacterial growth in contrast to 'KT-308' (Patel et al 2000.), whereas it could not provide more resistance to bacterial ingress compared to 'KT-308' or AH 26 (De Trey, Zurich, Switzerland; Padachey et al 2000). In another in vitro study, 'KT-308' effectively prevented penetration of E.faecalis into root canals, whereas 'ZUT' did not (McDougall et al 1999).

Resin-modified glass ionomer cements:

The most investigated RMGIC is vitrebond. Freshly mixed Vitrebond revealed a significant greater antimicrobial activity than the conventional cement Aquacem. The inhibitory properties were similar when the material was light cured or chemically cured. This suggests that antibacterial agents dissolved rapidly (Coogan & Crevan 1993). On one hand, it was suggested that the antibacterial activity was associated with low pH of the freshly mixed RMGIC combined with the release of fluoride ions above a threshold value. Furthermore, HEMA was also considered to contribute to the antimicrobial action. In case of Vitrebond, the marked antibacterial activity may be because of toxic agents released during curing, such as benzine bromine and benzine iodine (Geursten et al. 1998).

Adhesion

The adhesion of glass-ionomer cement sealer to the canal wall dentin has not been thoroughly investigated. Initial reports demonstrated close adaptation. Apparently, the interface of the sealer and the canal wall is influenced by the various endodontic irrigants and medicaments used prior to root filling. However, the nature of this influence is the subject of controversy. When the smear layer was removed, tags of the glass-ionomer cement were observed penetrating into the dentinal tubules, but to a lesser degree than with other sealers. Penetration of the filling material into the tubules is believed to improve the seal. Indeed, canals sealed with glass-ionomer cement after removal of the smear layer, demonstrated less leakage in vitro than those in which the smear layer was not removed. However, in other studies, removal of the smear layer did not appear to affect the seal. In fact, one study reported the seal was better with the smear layer present.

A recent investigation assessed that bond strength of two glass-ionomer cement sealers to bovine dentin conditioned with the common endodontic irrigants. The bond was weakest when the dentin was rinsed with 17% ethylene diaminetetraacetic acid (EDTA) to remove the smear layer. When the dentin was rinsed only with sodium hypochlorite, a hybrid layer was observed in the cement-dentin interface, which may have contributed to the strength of the bond.

The adhesion of GIC to dental tissue relies primarily on chemical interaction and, to a lesser extent, on micromechanical interlocking. Lalh et al (1999a) investigated the bond strength of two experimental GIC sealers ('KT-308' and 'ZUT') and Ketac-Endo to bovine dentin conditioned with the most common irrigants. Bond strength appeared to be lowest after treatment of dentin by 17% ethylene diamine tetra-acetic acid (EDTA) and 2.6% sodium hypochlorite. Irrigation with NaOCI or even with distilled water resulted in a higher bond strength and the formation of a hybrid layer between the GIC and the dentin. This research suggested that the smear layer should be preserved. In a more recent study (Timpavat t al 2001), contradictory results were obtained. Conditioning with phosphoric acid or citric acid, which was also more effective in removing the smear layer, resulted in higher bond strengts than conditioning with EDTA and NaOCI or conditioning with polyacrylic acid. According to this study, the smear layer should be removed. Aprt from this, Ketac-Endo demonstrated a lower shear bond strength than 'KT-308' or 'ZUT'.

Biocompatibility

Although it is widely accepted that glass-ionomer cement is biocompatible, several studies specifically assessed the biocompatibility of glass-ionomer cement sealers. In a comprehensive evaluation, Jonck et al. demonstrated excellent bone tolerance of experimental glass-ionomer cements, including a root canal sealer and a bone cement used in orthopedic surgery. The biocompatibility of the glass-ionomer sealer also was confirmed in the subcutaneous connective tissue.

Conventional GIC:

Research on the biocompatibility of GIC's in conventional and surgical endodontics has focused mainly on conventionally setting GIC's. The latter exhibit good biocompatibility for three main reasons (Nicholson et al.1991) i) set with minimum exotherm; ii) neutralizatio is generally sufficiently rapid that any potential irritation because of the presence of free acids is minimal; and iii) the substances leached from the set cement are generally either benign or beneficial to the tissue in which the cement is placed.

Crisp et al. (1978) measured setting exotherm and found that GICs gave the lowest setting exothermof any other biomedical cements and is a feature that contributes to the biocompatibility of GICs.

The species leached from a GIC are dependent on the initial constituents of the cement. Little or no organic species have been found to be lached out of GICs (Kuhn et al1983), the components described so far being all inorganic as follows:

Silica: The precise role of silica in the human metabolism is unclear, although it appears to lower the cholesterol levels in blood (Iler 1979). This, in combination with its low toxicity, suggests that the leaching of silica either in teeth or in bone is likely to be benign to the body.

Aluminium: In some respects, aluminium is the least biologically acceptable of all the leached elements. However, in endodontic applications, the release of aluminium would not be expected to cause problems. First, the amount released has been shown to be very small (Crisp et al. 1980, Brookman et al 1986); secondly, any release that occur, takes place in close proximity to mineralized tissues, either teeth or bone. The main constituent of this mineralized tissue is hydroxy-apatite, and because of its size, the AI^{3+} ion would be expected to occupy suitable vacancies in the surfaces of this material (Atkinson & Witt 1985).

Calcium: Is released in very small amounts (Crisp et al. 1980, Brookman et al 1986) and is beneficial to mineralized tissues. As the main inorganic content of teeth and bone is calcium phosphate mineral hydroxy-apatite, calcium can be incorporated in the hydroxy-apatite during remodeling of the bone (Atkinson & Witt 1985).

Phosphate: Ionomer glasses do not necessarily contain phosphate, although most of the commercially ones do. Its most useful physiological use is the formation of mineral hydroxy-apatite (Nicholson et al.1991).

Fluoride: The fluoride ions fit well than the hydroxyl ion into the hydroxy-apatite lattice of the teeth, which, afterwards, is more resistant to the attack of acids produced in the mouth (Atkinson & Witt 1985). The fluoride ions can be incorporated into the bone, which is less easily resorbed and does not undergo ion exchange as readily as nonfluoridated bone (Atkinson & Witt 1985).

Root canal sealer

One of the requirements of an ideal root canal sealer is that it should be non-irritating to the periapical tissues and should be compatible with the living connective tissue (Grossman 1982). Although specific research on GIC root canal sealer is limited, GICs in general are belived to be biocompatible. Subcutaneous implantation in rats caused a mild inflammatory reaction on the fifth day, which diminished progressively, when compared to a Zinc-oxide-eugenol based sealer, Tubli seal. Jonck et al conducted a series of experiments on baboon and humans: GICs were non-toxic in bulk, and allowed, as well as promoted, normal haemopoitic and osteoblastic activities on the cement surface. The cement had no inhibitory effect on bone tissue development and there was a total absence of fibrous tissue envelopment with the cement being effectively incorporated into the bone. Osteoblastic activity has also been demonstrated in cell cultures in the presence of Ketac-Endo (Snyder et al 1997)

Sealing material (perforation, root-end filling) in surgical endodontics

The use of GICs in the periradicular region implies that the material will have direct contact with the healing bone. Direct contact will takes place between the mineralized bone and root dentin, as well as the cementum (Craig & Harisson 1993, Torabinejad et al 1995). Bone implantation studies confirmed good tolerance to different kinds of GICs. Unfortunately, this interpretation of this bone implantation is difficult. However, more relevant clinical studies confirm the biocompatibility (Callis & Santini 1987, Zetterqvist et al. 1987).

Resin-modified glass ionomer cements

Resin modified glass ionomer cements contain unsaturated groups and hence may lack the biocompatibility of conventionally setting GICs, and concerns have been raised against their use. Moreover, differences in the amounts of fluoride released and cytotoxicity amongst RMGICs have been reported. Aluminium is also released from RMGICs in the short term, as well as long term. According to Geursten et al the eluetes in the RMGICs were the prime causes for cutotoxic reactions. The cytotoxicity of Vitremer has been studied (Yoshikawa et al. 1994, Kan et al 1998), and the release of HEMA has been shown to be one of the prime causes. Vitrebond used for pulp capping was more irritating to the pulp tissue than the calcium hydroxide. On the other hand, direct pulp capping with Vitremer did not seem to cause pulpal inflammation, and Vitremer im[lants only caused slight reactions in rabbits.

Compared to conventional GICs, RMGICs have easier handling properties: this, in association with their adhesion potential, makes them attractive as root-end filling materials. The low cytotoxicity and the pronounced antibacterial activity, as well as a favorable tissue response when used as a root-end filling material in the infected teeth, demonstrated that this material might be used in endodontic surgeries.

Clinical efficacy

To date, only one clinical study has been reported on the outcome of endodontic therapy using a glass-ionomer cement sealer. The results of this study were influenced by the nature of the cases treated, many of which had been complicated by a variety of factors known to lower the prognosis of treatment, and by the criteria used for assessment of the outcomes. Nevertheless, the reported rates of 78% success and only 6% failure are well within the range of those reported in many other studies in which conventional sealers were used. One of the observations in the clinical study was that the glass-ionomer cement persisted in the tissues when extruded periapically, in contrast to other sealers which are normally absorbed within a relatively short period of time. The persistence of the glass-ionomer sealer in the periradicular tissues confirms its very low tissue solubility, as well as its biocompatibility in the osseous environment.

Retrograde Root Canal Filling

A retrograde filling is placed to provide an apical seal in teeth with infected canals that cannot be accessed or negotiated coronally. Because the canal remains infected, the quality of the retrograde seal determines the outcome of the treatment. In this application, short working and setting times are not an impediment; in fact, they may be an advantage. Therefore, glass-ionomer cements used routinely for restorative applications were considered for retrograde filling long before a specific glass-ionomer sealer was developed. Consequently, studies have evaluated conventional glass-ionomer cements, as well as resin-based and silver-containing formulations. The main obstacle in the clinical application of glass-ionomers as retrograde filling materials is the difficulty of controlling the dryness of the surgical working field. On the other hand, in contrast to conventional cavity-retained retrograde fillings, the bonding of the glass-ionomer cement to the root dentin allows its application as a bonded cap over the resected root surface to improve the seal.

Sealing efficacy

Many in vitro studies have compared various formulations of glass-ionomer cement, with and without varnish, to other retrograde filling materials, mainly amalgam. Contradictions among these studies and the limitations of their methodologies do not warrant a clear conclusion; however, the overall performance of glass-ionomer cement in earlier leakage studies was better than that of other materials, with the exception of resin composite.

Several of the later studies also demonstrated minimal leakage with glass-ionomer retrograde fillings, particularly when it was applied in conjunction with varnish. Other studies failed to demonstrate a better seal with glass-ionomers, or even observed a poorer seal than that achieved with other materials. When the different formulations of glass-ionomer cement were compared with each other, the resin-modified material demonstrated a better seal than the conventional cement, and both were better than a silver-containing material.

Biocompatibility

When glass-ionomer cement is used as a retrograde filling, it is expected to come into direct contact with the healing alveolar bone, as opposed to when it is used as a restorative that interacts with the dentin, pulp, and gingiva. As healing takes place after apical surgery, deposition of mineralized tissue is expected to occur over the resected root surface and the retrograde filling. Accordingly, several studies have focused on the interaction between glass-ionomer cements and bone. From bone implantation studies, it appears that the different types of glass-ionomer cement are well tolerated by bone. However, the interpretation and correlation of results obtained in such studies is problematic. The more clinically relevant usage studies, in which functioning retrograde fillings interact with the surrounding tissues, also have confirmed the compatibility of glass-ionomer cement with bone.[75-78] Due to this compatibility, bone can grow directly over the glass ionomer, without an interface of connective or inflammatory tissue.

Clinical efficacy

Zetterqvist et al and later Jesslen et al also assessed the long-term outcome of apicoectomy relying on retrograde filling with glass-ionomer cement or amalgam. Using clinical and radiographic criteria to assess healing, these researchers demonstrated comparable results for the two materials. Thus, glass-ionomer cement proved to be an acceptable retrograde filling material, and it did not appear to be affected by the wet environment of surgery. Assessment of the clinical efficacy of a retrograde filling material in a clinical study is difficult due to multiple factors that may influence the outcome of the treatment. To minimize the variables, Friedman et al assessed the efficacy of retrograde filling materials in an animal model. The root canals, deliberately infected to induce periapical pathosis, were sealed by retrograde fillings and periapical healing was examined several months later. The reported performance of glass-ionomer cement in studies based on this model has been comparable to that of amalgam, but somewhat poorer than that of zinc oxide-eugenol cements. These results contrast the failure of glass-ionomer cement to seal infected canals in an earlier study.

Perforation Repair

Root perforation is an undesirable complication of root canal preparation and often leads to tooth extraction (Fuss & Trope 1996). Successful tretment depends on immediate sealing of the perforation and prevention of infection. In addition to factors related to the perforation itself, such as time elapsed since the perforation occurred and size & location of the perforation, the repair material is also of importance.

The prognosis of perforation repair depends primarily on the ability to eliminate the pathway of the periradicular infection. Secondary factors include the healing potential of the periradicular tissues, which is related to the duration of the perforation, its size and location, and the tissue compatibility of the repair material. Thus, the material used for perforation repair should possess good sealing, antimicrobial, and biocompatibility properties. The prevalence of perforations in endodontically treated teeth is under 10%. Because a variety of materials have been used for the repair of perforations, only limited information is available on the suitability and efficacy of glass-ionomer cements applied in this capacity.

Although of limited clinical relevance, several in vitro leakage studies have tested the seal of repaired perforations. With the exception of one study, they support the suitability of glass-ionomer cement for this application. Another in vitro study demonstrated the potential of a glass-ionomer root canal sealer to stimulate osteoblastic activity in cell culture. In a well-documented case report, Goon and Lundergan demonstrated the successful repair of a perforation with a glass-ionomer sealer after previous treatment attempts with gutta-percha and guided tissue regeneration had failed. Additional cases of successful perforation repair with glass-ionomer cement were reported by Fuss and Trope. From the reported cases it appears that glass-ionomer cement is well suited for perforation repair in a variety of clinical situations.

Clinical evaluation

Goon and Lundergan (1995), Shuman (1999), Behnia et al (2000), Breault et al (2000) described the successful repair of perforations with GIC. From these cases, GIC appeared to be a suitable material for repair of perforations or near perforations, where it acted as a substitute for dentin.

Repair of root resorption cavities

Through debridement and cleaning of the resorption cavity are essential for a good prognosis (Gutman & Harison 1994). Moreover, longterm success is also influenced by the use of a biocompatible restorative material (Demoor et al. 2002). As previously stated, because of the long setting reaction, hydration of GICs during the initial setting influences the longterm properties through contact with the moist environment. Nevertheless contemporary chemically cured GICs appear to perform well; Ketac-Fil used for the repair of resorption defects gave satisfactory results for atleast 4 years (Demoor et al 2002).

Glass-ionomer cement also can be applied over dentin in near perforation situations to prevent potential infection of the periradicular tissues. In these situations, the glass-ionomer cement substitutes for the lost dentin.

Treatment of Vertical Fractures

Vertical fractures occasionally occur in vital teeth, both intact and those with large restorations, because of excessive occlusal forces or traumatic injuries. In endodontically treated teeth, vertival fractures are more frequent. In a vertically fractured tooth, the fracture line becomes infected resulting in bone loss along the fracture line. Consequently, to successfully treat a fractured tooth and to eliminate the infection, the fracture line needs to be eliminated or, when a complete fracture is present, the tooth segments must be bonded together. A biocompatible environment should be maintained to obtain reattachment of periradicular tissues.

Repair attempts of vertically fractured teeth are rare. The pathogenic mechanism of vertical fractures is through the propagation of intraoral microorganisms and the resulting bone loss along the fracture line. Accordingly, treatment attempts should be directed toward the elimination of the fracture line as a pathway for microbial propagation, while maintaining a biocompatible environment for reattachment of the periradicular tissues. For teeth that are completely fractured, bonding the tooth segments together is an additional requirement.

The ability of glass-ionomers to bond split teeth is less than that of bonding agents and cyanoacrylate cement. However, due to its good biocompatibility, glass-ionomer cement has been considered the material of choice for filling the canals of treated fractured teeth, filling the fracture line, and repairing completely fractured teeth.

Stewart filled canals temporarily with calcium hydroxide to combat microorganisms and induce repair of the fracture line by deposition of cementum. After initial healing, the canals were filled with glass-ionomer cement. In the few cases treated in this manner, the teeth were retained for 2 to 10 years. Another approach to treatment involves a surgical intervention, during which the fracture line is filled. The few clinical cases reported on incompletely fractured teeth treated in this manner demonstrated a poor outcome for this procedure. At best, the teeth were retained for several months, even when treatment was combined with guided tissue regeneration.

Coronal Sealing After Root Canal Treatment

Even after completion of endodontic treatment, teeth are at risk of reinfection via ingress of microorganisms from the access cavity into the filled canals. The ability of the coronal restoration to prevent bacterial ingress is therefore one of the factors that influence the outcome of treatment. There are, however, specific considerations for the application of glass-ionomer cement in conjunction with the restoration of endodontically treated teeth.

To prevent bacterial ingress into the filled canals, the canal orifices and the floor of the pulp chamber in multirooted teeth can be sealed with a restorative material. Again, materials with good sealing properties are best suited for this application; accordingly, they are assessed by means of leakage studies in vitro. In one such study, glass-ionomer cement was found to be inferior to other materials. However, a barrier of resin-modified glass-ionomer cement was effective against microbial ingress into the canals.

In vitro evaluation:

Although there is no clinical evidence, GICs perform well as a coronal filling material in vitro compared to other materials. Placement of GIC in the canal orfices and on the floor of the pulp chamber of multi rooted teeth clearly diminished the ingress of microorganisms from the access cavity of the filled root canals. In one study, using the fluid filteration method, GIC microleakage values did not differ significantly from the intact crown values

Summary

Glass-ionomer cements have been used in endodontics for a variety of applications. Overall, they appear to be well suited for these uses, in which bone and soft tissue compatibility, sealing efficacy, and antimicrobial activity are more critical than tensile strength. Although the results of the numerous in vitro studies of glass- ionomer cement may appear diverse and inconclusive and the antimicrobial activity of glass-ionomer cement may not be optimal, clinical reports and well-designed animal studies have demonstrated acceptable clinical performance of this material in endodontic therapy.

13. CONCLUSION

Conclusion:

Since the development of glass-ionomer materials in the early 1970s, they have proved to be of value for the restoration of initial carious lesions, erosion/abrasion/ abfraction lesions, and the control of advancing caries, particularly where the occlusal load is not excessive. It is the only material presently available that can be regarded as bioactive, or therapeutic, because it has the potential for encouraging remineralization of surrounding tooth structure and has been shown to be bioactive in relation to bone. It also prevents bacterial microleakage because of the ion exchange adhesion that develops with both enamel and dentin. Glass-ionomer cement develops a new ion-enriched material at the interface with tooth structure, which consists of phosphate and calcium ions from enamel or dentin and calcium (or strontium), phosphate, and aluminum ions from the cement. It is interesting to note that in some materials the calcium in the glass has been replaced with strontium and, because strontium is also an apatite-forming specie, this has facilitated observation of the ion exchange phenomenon. If there is subsequent failure of a restoration, it occurs within cohesiveness of the glass-ionomer, leaving the ion exchange adhesion layer firmly attached to the cavity wall. This means that the dentinal tubules remain sealed against penetration of bacteria or their toxins.

Glass ionomers are available in acceptable esthetic forms, and resin modified materials are quite translucent. The physical properties of the latest autocured materials are close to those of microfilled resin composites, and the wear factor is not a problem once the material has matured. However, fracture resistance is a little lower than that of resin composite, meaning that, unless a restoration is well surrounded and supported by remaining natural tooth structure, it should be covered with another material (the "sandwich" technique) to provide the required strength and ensure longevity.

It is apparent that glass-ionomers have come of age and should be regarded as moderately biomimetic materials. The setting reaction, adhesion to tooth structure, and ion release remain the same, but the compressive and tensile strength are reduced because of a lower powder content in the mix.

Resin-modified luting cements are now available and these can also be used to bond amalgam to the cavity wall. Clinical observation has so far been limited, but research continues and there is no doubt their clinical uses will expand. Current investigations into the therapeutic benefits of glass-ionomers show considerable promise but the main limitation of these materials is low fracture resistance. If this can be improved, it is likely their uses will expand still further.

Meanwhile, glass-ionomer cements have reached the stage where they can be regarded as the trigger for the introduction of a far more conservative approach to the treatment of initial carious lesions. Either alone or in combination with resin composites, they make it possible to retain natural tooth structure to a far greater extent than before. The traditional surgical approach to the treatment of caries was dictated, in the absence of adhesion and fluoride, by the need to make room for the placement and condensation of amalgam and always resulted in a cavity that extended well beyond the confines of the lesion itself. All the parameters of this approach should now be abandoned, with preservation and remineralization of tooth structure becoming the driving force behind operative dentistry.

14. REFERENCES

1.Xie D, Park JG, Zhao J.Synthesis and preparation of novel 4-arm star shape poly(carboxylic acids)for improved light cure GICs.Dent Mater 2007; 23:395-403.

2. Mount GJ-Glass ionomer cements-an atlas.2nd ed United Kingdom:Martin Dunitz;1994.

3. Davidson CL. Advances in glass-ionomer cements J Appl Oral Sci. 2006;14:3-9

4. Wilson AD , Mclean JW. Glass-Ionomer Cement. Chicago, Quintessence Pub. Co.Int. 1992

5. Mclean JW. Evolution of Glass-Ionomer Cements: A Personal View. J Esthet Dent 1994; (6):195-206.
6. Suzuki M ,Jordan RE. Glass-Ionomer – Composite sandwitch technique. J Am Dent Assoc 1990; 120: 55-7.
7. Hunt PR. Microconservative restorations for approximal carious lesions. J Am Dent Assoc 1990; 120: 37-40
8. Mclean JW. Cermet Cements. J Am Dent Assoc 1990; 120: 43-7.
9. Simmons J J. Silver alloy powder & Glass Ionomer Cement. J Am Dent Assoc 1990; 120: 49-52
10. Smith DC. Composition & characteristics of Glass Ionomer Cements. J Am Dent Assoc 1990; 120:20-3
11. Wilson AD. Developments in Glass Ionomer Cements. Int J Prosthodont 1989;2:438-46
12. Crisp S ,Wilson AD. Reactions in glass inomer cements v. effect of incorporating tartaric acid in the cement forming liquid. J Dent Res 1976; 55: 1023-31.
13. Mclean JW. Clinical applications of Glass Ionomer Cements. Oper Dent 1992;5: 184-90
14. Albers. Tooth Colored Restorative Cements 9th ed.London;BcDecker:2002.
15. Croll TP , Nicholson JW. Glass Ionomer Cements in pediatric dentistry. Pediatr Dent 2002;24:423-29
16. WWW.GC Fuji Asia.com
17. Frankenberger R,Sindel J. Viscous Glass Ionomer Cements: A new Alternative to amalgam in the primary dentition. Quintessence Int 1997; 28: 667-76
18. Christenson GJ. Glass Ionomer as luting cement. J Am Dent Assoc 1990; 120: 59-62
19. Hse K M Y, Leung S K, Wei S H Y. Resin – ionomer restorative materials for children: review. Aust Dent J 1999;44: 1-11.
20. Mount GJ. Glass-ionomer cements: Past, present, and future. Oper Dent 1994;19:82-90.
21. Mount GJ. Glass-ionomers: A review of their current status. Oper Dent 1999;24: 115-23.
22. Yelamanchili A,Darvell W. Network competition in a RMGIC Dent Mater 2008; 1065-69.

23. Vaikuntam J. Resin modified glass ionmer cements: implications for use in pediatric dentistry. J dent for child; 1997: 131-34
24. SidhuK.S Clinical evaluations of resin modified glass ionomer restorations. Dent Mater.2010 ;26;:7-12.

25. Combe C & Douglass WH. The future of dental materials. Dent update 1998;25:412-17
26. John F,McCABE, Zhuoqun YAN, Omar T, Mahmoud M ,Sarah L. R. Smart materials in dentistry – future prospects. Dent Mater J 2009; 28(1): 37 – 43
27. Brook IM, Hatton PV. Glass Ionomers: Bio Active Implant Materials. Biomaterials. 1998; 19:5-20.
28. Yap AU.Experimental studies on a new bioactive material: HAIonomer cements. Biomaterials. 2002;23:955-62.
29. Khara MK. Effect of polyacrylic acid on the apatite formation of a bioactive ceramic in a simulated body fluid: fundamental examination of the possibility of obtaining bioactive glass-ionomer cements for orthopaedic use. Biomaterials 2001;22:3191-6.
30. Urpo H, Narhi M, Narhi T. Compound changes and tooth mineralization effects of glass ionomer cements containing bioactive glass (S53P4) Biomaterials 2005; 26:5934-41.
31. Ikemura K,Tay FR,Endo T,Pashley SH. A Review of Chemical-approach and Ultramorphological Studies on the Development of Fluoride-releasing Dental Adhesives Comprising New Pre-Reacted Glass Ionomer (PRG) Fillers. Dent. Mater. J. 2008; 27(3): 315-39
32. Urpo H et al. Release of silica, calcium, phosphorus, and fluoride from glass ionomer cement containing bioactive glass. J of Biomater Appl 2004; 19:565-71.
33. Yap AUJ, Tham SY, Zhu LY, Lee HK. Short-term fluoride release from various aesthetic restorative materials. Oper Dent 2002;27:259-265.
34. Hoszek . Chlorhexidine Containing Glass Ionomer Cement. Swed Dent J 2005;29:89-96.
35. Turkun LS. Long term antibacterial effects of Chx containing GIC. J.Esthet. Restorative.Dent.20:29-45 2008
36. Sanders BJ . Resin modified glass-ionomers combined with Chlorhexidine. J Oral Rehabil 2002;29:553-8.
37. Feilzer AJ, Kakaboura AI, De Gee AJ, Davidson CL. The influence of water sorption on the developments of setting shrinkage stress in traditional and light curing glass-ionomer cements. Dent Mater 1995;11 :186-190.
38. Stamboulis A , Matsuya S , Hill RG , Law RG ,Udoh K ,Nakagawa M et.al .MAS-NMR spectroscopy studies in the setting reaction of glass ionomer cements.J Dent 2006;5:574 - 8 1
39. Nicholson JW,Czarneka B.The biocompatibility of resin-modified glass ionomer cements for dentistry.Dent Mater 2008 Dec;24(12):1702-8.
40. Meşe.A,Burrow.M.F,Tyas.M.J Sorption and solubility of luting cements in different solutions. Dent Mater J 2008; 27(5): 702 – 709
41. Van Meerbeek B, Willems G, Celis JP, Roos JR, Braem M, Lambrechts P, Vanherle G. Assessment by nano-indentation of the hardness and elasticity of the resin-dentin bonding.J Dent Res 1993;72:1434-42
42. GeeDe AJ, Duinen RNB, Werner A,Davidson CL. Early & Long Term Wear Of Conventional & Resin-Modified Glass Ionmers .J Dent Res 1996;75(8): 1613-19.

43. Huysmann MC,Vander Varst PGT,Schafer R,Peters MC.Fatigue behavior of restorative aterials,Dent.Mater 1995;11:137-41.
44. Shen C, Grimaudo N. Effect of hydration on the biaxial flexural strength of a glass-ionomer cement. Dent Mater 1994;10:190-5.
45. Jevnikar P, Jarh, Sepe A, Pintar MM, Funduk M N. Micro magnetic resonance imaging of water uptake by glass-ionomer cements. Dent Mater 1997; 13:20-3.
46. De Moore RGJ, Veerbek RM. Fluoride release profile of restorative glass-ionomer formulations Dent Mater 1996;12:88-95.
47. Marczuk,Kolada G. – Fluoride release and antibacterial activity of selected GICs.Postepy Hig Med Dosw. (online), 2006; 60: 416-20
48. Forss H. The release of fluoride and other elements from light-cured glass-ionomers in neutral and acidic conditions. J Dent Res 1993;72: 1257-62.
49. El-Mallakh B, Sarkar NK. Fluoride releae from glass-ionomer cements in de-ionized water & artificial saliva. Dent Mater 1990;6: 118-122.
50. Tam LE, Chan GP, Vim D. In vitro caries inhibition effects by conventional and resin modified glass-ionomer restorations. Oper Dent 1997;22:4-14.
51. Tsanidis V, Koulourides T. An in vitro model for assessment of fluoride uptake from glass-ionomer cements by dentin and its effect on acid resistance. Dent Res 1992;71: 7-12.
52. Forss H, Nase L, Seppa L. Fluoride concentration, mutans streptococci and lactobacilli in plaque from old glass-ionomer fillings. Caries Res 1995;29:50-3.
53. Loyola-rodriguez JP, Garcia godoy F. Growth inhibition of glass ionomer cements on Mutans Streptococci. Pediatr Dent 1994; 16:346-9
54. Markovic DL, Petrovic BB and Peric TO. Fluoride content and recharge ability of five glassionomer dental materials. BMC Oral Health 2008, **8**:21.
55. Erickson RL. Elemental analysis of artificial caries lesions adjacent to fluoride releasing materials. J Dent Res 1995;74:440.
56. Ten Cate JM, van Duinen RN. Hyper- Mineralization of dentinal lesions adjacent to glass-ionomer cement restoration. J Dent Res 1995; 74:1266-71.
57. Rezk-Lega F, Jgaard , Arends J. An in vivo study on the merits of two glass-ionomers for the cementation of orthodontic bands. Am J Orthod Dentofacial Orthop 1991 ;99:162-7.
58. Kakaboura A, Papagiannoulis L, Eliades G. In vitro vs in vivo anticariogenic potential of esthetic restorative materials. J Dent Res 1998;77:658.
59. Hien C,Mount GJ, Intyre JM , Tuisuva J , Doussa RJV. Chemical exchange between glass-ionomer restorations and residual carious dentine in permanent molars:An in vivo study. J Dent 2006; 608-13.
60. Mônica T, Antônio A, Guedes C, Chevitarese PO. Braz Oral Res 2006;20(2):91-6
61. Meerbeek BV, Inokoshi S, Braem M, Lambrechts P, Vanherle G. Morphological aspects of the resin-dentin interdiffusion zone with different dentin adhesive systems. J Dent Res 1992; 71: 1530-40.

62. Orbans. Oral Histology. 12 ed.India;Elsevier:2006.
63. Ten Cate R. Oral Histology: Development, Structure and Function.6th ed.Missouri;Mosby:2006
64. Briso ALF, Rahal V, Mestrener SR,Dezan EJ. Biological response of pulps submitted to different capping materials. Braz Oral Res 2006;20(2):91-6.
65. Kan KC, Messer LB. Variability in cytotoxicity & fluoride release of resin modified glass ionomer cements. J Dent Res1997; 76: 1502-07.
66. Nicholsan JW,Czarnecka B; The biocompatibility o resin modified GICs for dentistry.dental materials.2008;24:1702-08.
67. Modena KCL. Cytotoxicity and biocompatibility of direct and indirect pulp capping materials. J Appl Oral Sci. 2009;17(6):544-54.
68. Hatton PV, Hurrell K,Gillingham, Brook IM,Biocompatibility of glass-ionomer bone cements. J Dent; 2006(34) 598 –60.
69. Gillingham KH , Reaney IM, Brook I , Hatton PV , In vitro biocompatibility of a novel Fe2O3 based glass ionomer cement, J Dent 2006 ;34: 53 3 – 53
70. Mount GJ. Adhesion of glass-ionomer cement in the clinical environment. Oper Dent 1991 ; 16: 141-8.
71. Czarnecka B,Nicholson JW.Ion release by resin-modified glass-ionomer cements into water and lactic acid solutions, J Dent; 2006;34:608-13.
72. McLean JW. Dentinal bonding agents versus glass-ionomer cements. Quintessence Int 1996; 27:659-67.
73. Scholte CM, Davidson CL. Complete marginal seal of class V resin composite restorations effected by increased flexibility. J Dent Res 1990;69:1240-43.
74. Davidson CL. Glass-ionomer bases under posterior composites. J Esthet Dent 1994; 6:223-26.
75. Johnson GH, Powel LV, Derouen TA. Evaluation and control of post-cementation pulpal sensitivity: Zinc phosphate and Glass-Ionomer luting cements. J Am Dent Assoc 1993; 124:39-46.
76. Mitra SB, Kedrowski BL. Long-term mechanical properties of glass-ionomers. Dent Mater 1994;19:78-82.
77. Reinhardt JW, Swift EJ Jr, Bolden AJ. A national survey on the use of glass-ionomer cements. Oper Dent 1993;18:56-60.
78. Christensen GJ. Why is glass ionomer cement so popular? J Am Dent Assoc 1994;125: 1257-58.
79. Mitra SB. Adhesion to dentin and physical properties of a light-cured glass-ionomer liner/base. J Dent Res 1991;70:72-74.
80. Friedl KH, Schmalz G, Hiller KA, Geismeier R, Lang P. Bond strength of hybrId ionomer and compomer luting materials. J Dent Res 1998;77:814.
81. Kakaboura A, Eliades G, Palaghias G. An FTIR study on the setting mechanism of resin-modified glass-ionomer restoratives. Dent Mater 1996; 12:173-178.

82. Gladys S,Meerbeek V ,Braem M,Lambrechts P,Vanherle G. Comparative physico-mechanical characterization of new hybrid restorative materials with conventional glass-ionomer and resin composite restorative materials. J Dent Res 1997;76:883-94
83. Tan K, Lim CC, Chan YM. The effect of resin and resin-ionomer cements on crown seating. J Dent Res 1998;77:925 [abstract 2347].
84. Fritz UB, Finger WJ, Uno S. Resin-modffied glass-ionomer cements: Bonding to enamel and dentin. Dent Mater 1996;12:161-166.
85. Syrek A. Features of modern GICs and their relevance to clinical practice. J Dent. 2006;34(8):614-22.
86. Swift EJ, Lloyd AH, Felton DA. The effect of resin desensitizing agents on crown retention. J Am Dent Assoc 1997;128:195-200.
87. Komori A, Ishikawa H. Evaluation of a resin- reinforced glass ionomer cement for use as an orthodontic bonding agent. Angle Orthod 1997;67:189-96.
88. Ogaard B, Arends J, Helseth H, Dijkman G, Van der Kuiji M. Fluoride level in saliva after bonding orthodontic brackets with a fluoride-containing adhesive. Am J Orthod Dentofacial Orthop 1997; 111 :199-202.
89. De Bruyne M A A & De Moor R J G. The use of glass ionomer cements in both conventional & surgical endodontics. Inter Endod J 2004;37:91-104.
90. Stewart GG. Clinical application of glass ionomer cements in endodontics: case reports. Inter Endod J 1990;23: 172-78.
91. Croll TP. Glass ionomers for infants, children and adolescents. J Am Dent Assoc 1990; 120:65-68.
92. Kennedy DB, Roberts JF, Curzon MEJ. Kennedy's pediatric operative dentistry.4th ed.Oxford;John Wright & sons:2004.
93. Christensen GJ. Restoration of pediatric posterior teeth. J Am Dent Assoc 1966; 127;
94. Francisconi LF,Scaffa PMC,Barros VP, Coutinho M, Francisconi PAS.Glass ionomer cements and their role in the restoration of non-carious cervical lesions. J. Appl. Oral Sci. vol.17 2009
95. Mount GJ. Longevity in glass-ionomer restorations: Review of a successful technique. Quintessence Int 1997; 28:643-50.
1. Hickel R, VoB A. A comparison of glass cermet cement and amalgam restorations in primary molars. J Dent child 1990; 57; 184.
97. Morand JM, Jonas P. Resin-modified glass- ionomer cement restoration of posterior teeth with proximal carious lesions. Quintessence Int 1995; 26:389-94.
98. Trachtenberg F,Maserjian N N,Socini J A,Hayes C,Taveres M.Does Flouride in Compomers prevent future caries in children.J Dent Res 2009;88:276-9.
99. Irie M,Suzuki K.Marginal seal of RMGIC:Effect of delaying polishing procedure after one day storage.Oper Dent 2000;25:488-96.
100. Hubel S,Mejare I.Conventional versus resin modified glass ionomer cement for Class II restorations in primary molars.A 3 year clinical study.Int J Pediatr Dent 2003;13:2-8.

101. Kramer N,Frankerberger R.Compomers in restorative therapy of children:A literature review.Int J Pediatr Dent 2007;17:2-9.
102. De bruyne M A,De Moore R J. The use of glass ionomers in both conventional and surgical endodontics.Int Endod J 2004;37:97-104.

Kolibri 360 GmbH
Ferdinand-Jühlke-Straße 7
99095 Erfurt, Deutschland
produktsicherheit@kolibri360.de

Druck:
CPI Druckdienstleistungen GmbH
im Auftrag der
Kolibri 360 GmbH
Ferdinand-Jühlke-Str. 7
99095 Erfurt